RIDE STRONG

RIDE STRONG

Essential Conditioning for Cyclists

Jo McRae

B L O O M S B U R Y

LONDON • OXFORD • NEW YORK • NEW DELHI • SYDNEY

Bloomsbury Sport
An imprint of Bloomsbury Publishing Plc

50 Bedford Square	1385 Broadway
London	New York
WC1B 3DP	NY 10018
UK	USA

www.bloomsbury.com

First published 2016

© Jo McRae, 2016
Illustrations by Dave Saunders and Louise Turpin, 2016
Photography: Hamish Brown (internal); Robin Bell (contents page and pp.286–87)

British Library Cataloguing-in-Publication Data
A catalogue record for this book is available from the British Library.

Library of Congress Cataloguing-in-Publication data has been applied for.

ISBN: PB: 978-1-4729-2860-3
       ePDF: 978-1-4729-2862-7
       ePub: 978-1-4729-2861-0

2 4 6 8 10 9 7 5 3 1

Typeset in Adobe Caslon Pro by seagulls.net
Printed and bound in China by Toppan Leefung Printing

To find out more about our authors and books visit www.bloomsbury.com. Here you will find extracts, author interviews, details of forthcoming events and the option to sign up for our newsletters.

Contents

Acknowledgements

I would like to acknowledge the importance of what I have learned through the CHEK institute in enabling me to write this book. Much of what I apply in my work with cyclists is an amalgamation of learning, but I rely on the knowledge I have gained through the CHEK institute the most.

I would like to thank my exercise models: Paul Callahan, Jake Martin and Nichola Roberts, who bring the book to life with the bodies of real cyclists. This makes the exercises all the more relevant and meaningful.

Hamish Brown has provided the stunning photographs that illustrate this book. I would like to thank Hamish for his support on this book as an artistic project. Thanks also to Robin Bell for allowing me to use his picture of Paul riding from Lands End to John O'groats on the contents page.

Most of all I would like to thank my close friends and family who have helped me take this book through its various incarnations to final completion. You know who you are. THANK YOU.

About the author and contributors

Jo McRae is a lifelong cyclist whose experience crosses a range of disciplines at national level competition with road racing, criteriums, time-trialling, track and cyclo-cross. She started racing bikes as a young girl, and having graduated from Loughborough University with a first class degree in sports science in 1998, she briefly represented Great Britain on the road in Australia before racing for a season in France supported by the Dave Rayner Fund.

On her return in 1999, Jo found work in the fitness industry exploring all avenues of teaching and training to build some real-world experience on top of her academic knowledge. Over the past 15 years she has developed a skill base that allows her to bridge the gaps between rehab, fitness and performance – merging several fields that otherwise have operated in isolation – and provide exercise programmes that meet the needs of the individual across the spectrum.

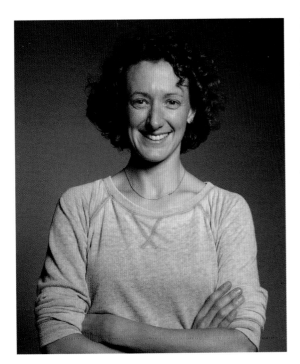

In recent years she has brought this knowledge back home and applied it to cyclists, specializing in providing off-the-bike conditioning programmes that dovetail with a rider's cycling training to maximize gains in performance and to minimize risk of injury.

Jo continues to ride regularly herself, but it's the challenge of getting the best out of other riders in her role as coach and mentor that she enjoys most.

You will see her throughout the book making adjustments to the models in Chapters 2, 3 and 4 as they work through the exercises.

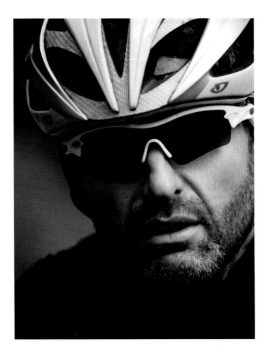

Paul Callahan is a weekend warrior and family man in his 40s who enjoys riding his bike to stay fit, to commute, and to get outside. He has dabbled in a bit of road racing and done a few time trials but mostly enjoys riding for the fun of it. In 2014 he rode from Land's End to John o' Groats with eight others, raising money for the Teenage Cancer Trust. He says of the journey: 'It was the ride of a lifetime, riding until sunset on an unknown path, making great friends and memories along the way.' The photo on the contents page shows Paul on that epic ride. He has promised to one day repeat the route with his wife, Tosie.

Paul illustrates the essential stretching exercises in Chapter 2. These are the most relevant for riders like him who benefit most from flexibility work.

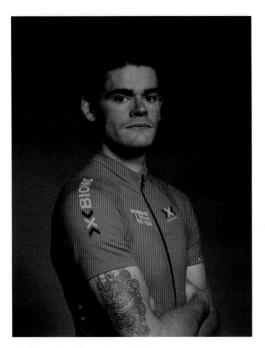

Jake Martin is a young (almost) full-time cyclist competing at national level in the UK at the time of writing. In recent years Jake has been trying to make a name for himself on the tough UK circuit. 2014 was a difficult season for Jake and his body shows the scars of the many crashes and injuries he sustained throughout that year in our photo shoot.

Jake illustrates the essential strength exercises in Chapter 3. These exercises are most relevant for riders looking to develop that extra edge in their performance and training and are willing to work consistently year round to gain the benefits.

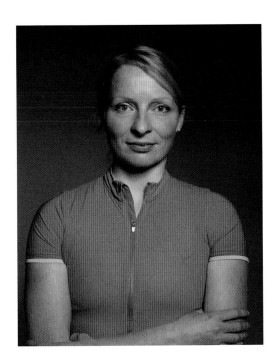

Nichola Roberts started competitive life late as a triathlete. After a cycling incident in 2012 prevented her running and swimming, she focused solely on cycling and has not looked back. She has competed in road racing to Cat 2, completed the Haute Route Pyrenees in 2013, finished first woman at Ride London, and has competed in various European Gran Fondos. Mostly, though, she cycles for the love of it and is never happier than when lost in the country lanes of Britain or the mountains of Europe.

Combining her passion for cycling with her profession as a physiotherapist, Nichola set up Velophysio in order to help people interrupted by injury to achieve their cycling goals. With 15 years' experience of working as a physiotherapist on sports injuries, together with specialist training in cycling, Nichola has found her calling.

Nichola illustrates the essential core exercises in Chapter 4. These exercises are most relevant for women and those with 'instability issues'. She demonstrates the 'more flexible' examples of stretches to contrast with the 'stiffer' examples given by Paul in Chapter 2, and also appears in the strength exercises in Chapter 3 with Jake.

Introduction

One of the best things about riding a bike is that it reminds us what it feels like to be a kid.

It gives us back the sense of pleasure and play that can be lost because of the pressures of modern life and being a grown-up. A bicycle can take us to amazing places, both physically and metaphorically. And often a reintroduction to the bike can kick-start a love affair with health and fitness too.

But I have some bad news that I want to get up front straight away. In many ways the human body is not designed to ride a bike.

The good news is that this book will give you the understanding and know-how to keep you riding your bike happily and healthily long into the future.

Even better, the same fundamental approach can make you a stronger, fitter cyclist. It will make you more able to climb hills, more able to cover long distances comfortably, and more able to sprint when the mood takes you. The exercises contained in this book will keep you problem free *and* allow you to reach your cycling potential within the time you have to exercise. I have written this book because this is what I want from my cycling, and because I know you want it too.

About this book

In writing this book I have had to make some generalizations about the likely readership, but just because I have taken a broad approach it doesn't mean that the information here is general. Each exercise has been carefully selected based on my knowledge and understanding of cycling, how the body works (and doesn't work) and more than a decade of experience working in health, fitness and sport.

This book is written for keen amateur road cyclists who work full-time and cycle for fun and fitness, or semi-competitively in races or sportives. The concepts outlined here are most relevant to 'time-poor' cyclists who perhaps ride between 6 and 14 hours a week and are looking for efficient ways to improve and enhance their performance and avoid pain and injury problems.

This book is written for both men and women, for the most part between the ages of 25 and 55. If I wrote a book specifically for women, for younger riders, or for older riders, there would be some differences in the exercises, but much of what I have to say here would still be relevant and useful.

For women reading this book, everything here still applies to you, but you are likely to find the 'strength' and 'core' exercise sections the most important. For most men in the upper end of this age bracket, starting with the stretches alone will give you enormous benefits.

Either way, for both male and female readers I would advise that you follow the basic principles outlined later by prioritizing flexibility first, then looking to improve your core control, before finally moving on to some more 'integrated' strength work. As is often the case, the exercises that you find the hardest will probably be the ones that you need the most. Chapter 6 on planning and periodization will help you find the right balance of exercises to meet your personal needs.

What will I need to get the most out of this book?

To maximize the benefits you will need a willingness to try some of the exercises yourself, and this will probably mean purchasing a 'Swiss ball' (gym ball), some foam rollers, some light dumbbells for use at home, and a yoga strap or martial arts belt to help with the hamstrings stretches. 'Spin lock' dumbbells that allow you to increase or decrease the weight by adding or removing small discs are the most convenient for at-home use as they take up the least space. A dimple dowel rod or broomstick handle can also come in useful for some of the exercises, as you will see later on.

I use Swiss balls a lot in my exercise programming because I find them to be a simple and versatile tool for home-based stretching, core and strengthening exercises. The exercises in this book are simple and straightforward, and I have pitched them at a level I feel you will be able to master on your own by following the instructions given. Don't let fear of 'doing them wrong' stop you from giving them a try.

For Swiss balls, AOK 'Duraballs' are the best on the market. In general the better the ball, the more you pay, but it's worth getting a good one. Check the ball you are using is burst-resistant and can withstand a user weight of 400kg. Your ball should not 'sag' when you sit on it and start to exercise with it, even with added weight.

As a size guide, most women will need a 55cm diameter ball (height 5'1–5'7") while most men will need a 65cm diameter ball (5'7"–6'2"). For those over 6'2" a 75cm ball may be considered, but a 65cm ball is often adequate and more practical because of the storage space needed for the larger ball.

If you feel inclined to progress further with the strengthening elements in particular, you may want to consider joining a gym or working with a trainer like myself on a more challenging or personalized programme. However, I have chosen the exercises in this book both for their effectiveness and also because you will be able to do them at home by yourself with very little equipment. For many cyclists, gym membership is unappealing for a number of reasons, so the Swiss ball offers a cheap and effective tool that bridges the gap between rehab (or 'prehab') and fitness where most everyday cyclists need to start.

Quick equipment checklist

- 4-inch-diameter foam roller, 35 inches in length, or longer for very tall people
- 6-inch-diameter foam roller, 25 inches long is adequate
- Tennis/cricket ball
- Swiss ball/stability ball
- Martial arts belt or yoga strap, non-elastic
- Spinlock dumbbells (York ones are widely available)
- A stick as a technique training tool and for support with some of the strength exercises

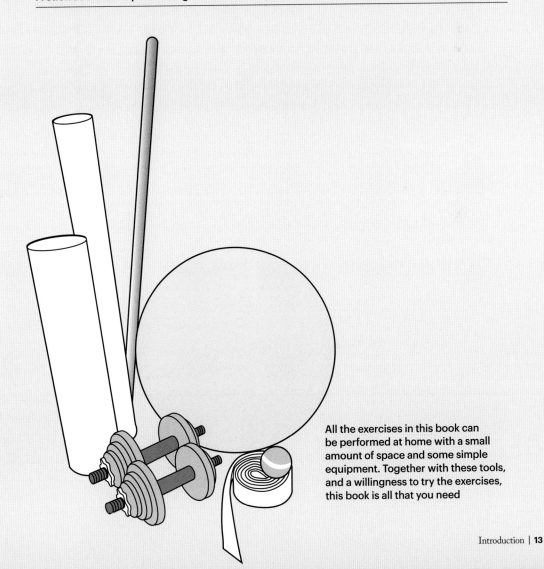

All the exercises in this book can be performed at home with a small amount of space and some simple equipment. Together with these tools, and a willingness to try the exercises, this book is all that you need

What this book isn't

Although I mention and discuss common injuries and issues associated with cycling in this book, it is not a substitute for 'treatment' of any of the injury problems discussed.

If you are in pain and are looking for ways to alleviate that pain then I suggest you see a physiotherapist, osteopath or remedial/sports masseur/therapist, depending on the nature of the problem.

Then when you are out of the 'acute' phase of the injury you can start to build a stronger, more resilient body using the exercises in this book to prevent the problem recurring.

In Chapter 4 on essential strength exercises I am acutely aware that I am only touching on a huge subject area and introducing the very basics to make a start.

If you are keen to develop your strength as much as possible then you may want to seek out a strength and conditioning coach (UKSCA) to maximize your progress.

How to use this book

I would love for you to read this book from cover to cover and digest its contents thoroughly. However, I am a realist and would like you to glean something useful from it even if you find yourself dipping in and out over coffee after a weekend ride. For the browser, I have highlighted key points throughout the text in a bolder font.

CHAPTER 1 of the book explains the background thinking behind my approach, giving the chosen exercises some context and **illustrating why I have selected the exercises in this book**. I will introduce you to the idea of the 'primal patterns' and why they should provide a framework for strength training for any cyclist – to prevent injury and enhance performance.

CHAPTERS 2, 3 and 4 are practical explanations of essential stretching, strength and core exercises, because more than anything I want you to *try* a handful of these so that you can immediately feel the benefits. There is nothing more compelling and motivating than noticing a difference straight away when you hit on an exercise that targets your weak spot. For this reason **I have listed the exercises at the start of each section in these chapters, so that you can quickly scan through and find what you are looking for.** For example, if you want to learn how to stretch your hamstrings because you know they are tight, you can go to the index for the 'essential stretching' in Chapter 2 and go straight to the stretch you need. **I have also included a 'ready reference' of thumbnail pictures of the exercises at the end of each of these chapters to help jog your memory as you work through them.**

CHAPTER 5 will cover some general **cross-training principles** and **highlight why some forms of exercise are complementary to your conditioning.** Once again, the index will list the topics so you can go straight to the mode of exercise you have in mind. For example, if you are thinking of running in the winter as a form of cross-training, you can look it up in the index and go straight there.

CHAPTER 6 will explain **how to design and periodize your own programme to create a year-round training plan** dovetailing all the elements in the book with your cycling season to maximize your gains in fitness. The emphasis of your programme will likely change throughout your season, so the balance of stretch, strength and core exercises is likely to be different depending on where you are in relation to your goals.

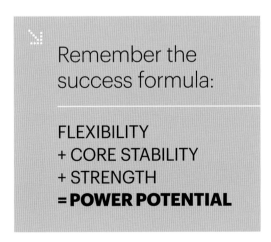

Remember the
success formula:

FLEXIBILITY
+ CORE STABILITY
+ STRENGTH
= POWER POTENTIAL

1. Body meet bike

 ## Overview of this chapter

Cycling in the context of human movement

In health and fitness circles the notion of 'primal' fitness has gained momentum over the last decade, with the key concept being that we have evolved to move through certain 'primal movement patterns' on a daily basis to maintain our physical potential.

In this chapter I am going to outline what these basic human movements are and their relevance to cyclists. Later, in Chapter 3 on essential strength exercises, I will give you some practical ways to train with these movements yourself.

This notion of primal fitness may seem like just another trend to some, but it is this simple but fundamental idea that forms the foundation of my approach to conditioning the body for the bike. It may seem counter-intuitive, but understanding our bodies in terms of our essential movement needs provides a solid conditioning platform upon which our cycling fitness can be built, pain and injury free, and with the greatest potential for optimal performance.

Two feet good, two wheels bad

The simplest and most obvious example of how our day-to-day movement has become 'unnatural' as we have modernized can be seen in how we get from A to B. The human body has spent thousands of years evolving a specialist movement pattern for that purpose. Collectively termed 'gait', our ability to walk, jog and run upright is what makes us unique among the animal kingdom. The human spine is especially adapted for being upright, and its curvatures have developed to facilitate our physical function.

We have an inward curve at the lower back (the lumbar lordosis), an outward curve at the upper back (thoracic kyphosis), and an inward curve at the neck (cervical lordosis). The discs between the lumbar vertebrae assist with cushioning against load, and the shape of the thoracic vertebrae facilitates rotation and maximizes mobility. These curves of the spine, together with its rotation as we walk and move, makes human gait extremely efficient and specialized, with our opposing arm swing adding to the movement via the connective tissue of the core (Gracovetsky, 1988).

In contrast to this remarkably evolved and uniquely human movement, when we swing our leg over a bike and sit in the saddle we are using engineering and mechanical efficiency *through* the bicycle to aid our movement. We have effectively used our highly evolved brain to create a machine that can get us from A to B even quicker. The engineering masterpiece of the bicycle is the triumph of the human brain over the limitations of our physical body, offering us many benefits not only for transport but also for sport and leisure.

 # Body, meet bike

And so we come to a fundamental human truth; we evolved to walk the earth, not pedal it. And although the invention of the bicycle has given us both a useful method of transport and a fun gadget to play with, taking on board this basic biomechanical fact can help ensure that your cycling has a wholly positive impact on your health and well-being and doesn't come with any negative side effects. Understanding how the body is designed to move can help you not only stay injury free, but also perform at your best by way of maintaining flexibility and strength parameters that translate to fitness and power on the bike.

If cycling becomes your only means of exercise in an otherwise sedentary lifestyle, you can encounter problems, and in this chapter I am going to explain why.

Providing structure, movement and support to the human body, **the musculoskeletal system** is a term given to the muscles and bones together. Although most musculoskeletal problems are not immediately life threatening, they can significantly affect your quality of life and ability to exercise. Consequently, your musculoskeletal health underpins your ability to move without pain or injury and your potential for optimal physical performance as a cyclist.

Aside from aches and pains caused by impact injuries, most recurrent niggles are chronic problems caused by changes in muscle length, and subsequent loss of joint mobility and core control. These issues have often taken some time to develop and therefore can take some time to unravel. By the time we have a symptom or 'pain' we may be at a tipping point where treatment alone provides only temporary relief and where taking a proactive and considered approach with exercise is essential in order to prevent the problem from worsening.

It's true that cycling is 'kind' to the body as an exercise option, because it's 'low impact' – which is why many people turn to cycling in the first place. But recurrent muscle or joint problems can stop you riding your bike, something any keen cyclist fears the most. An enforced break from the bike can be inconvenient and depressing, and so learning to protect and nurture your musculoskeletal health is essential if you want to continue riding uninterrupted by common problems.

Sitting culture, seated sports

Even the low impact nature of cycling can become a negative influence in the long run for a body designed to have feet making regular contact with the ground. With a well-aligned body and upright spine, the ground forces coming up through the feet as we walk, run and move are a positive stimulus, transmitting force through the springlike mechanisms of the fascia (tissues surrounding and linking the muscles), stimulating positive bone density changes and creating a natural pumping mechanism for the viscera or internal organs, keeping them healthy and mobile.

Seated on a bicycle our spinal alignment is very different to our upright walking posture. The lumbar curve is reversed, maintaining a flexed position, and the upper back does not rotate and move in its normal manner. In order for us to be able to see where we are going the neck has an excessive inward curve as we look forwards and ahead of us. These deviations from the human 'norm' can cause problems when this posture is often repeated without any 'corrective' or 'balancing' measures to counter the time spent in the saddle.

Our position on a bike as a posture for prolonged movement represents a significant deviation from the biomechanical or primal 'norm' of upright walking, jogging or running.

In addition to the potential problems caused by cycling itself, most of us now spend an inordinate amount of our time sitting in a chair, another modern shift that negates our evolutionary resting postures such as kneeling, squatting and sitting cross-legged. Under more 'primitive' conditions these postures represent an important part of our movement vocabulary and would have helped to keep joints mobile and muscles long.

Our office-based work culture has long been recognized as problematic for back health, and with 'work' now being largely cerebral rather than physical we are encouraged to get our exercise as part of our leisure. While cycling has the advantage of allowing us the freedom to roam in the fresh air as we raise our heart rate, it does not offer the body all of its biological movement requirements.

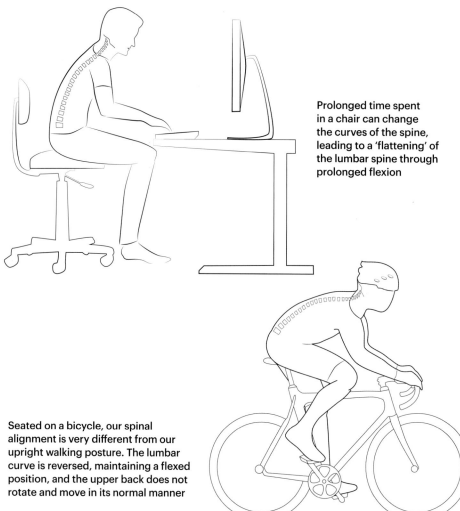

An upright posture and a neutral spine represents the normal human position to move from, supporting the spring like mechanisms of the spine, and providing a start position for the primal patterns

Prolonged time spent in a chair can change the curves of the spine, leading to a 'flattening' of the lumbar spine through prolonged flexion

Seated on a bicycle, our spinal alignment is very different from our upright walking posture. The lumbar curve is reversed, maintaining a flexed position, and the upper back does not rotate and move in its normal manner

Where a seated lifestyle can cause problems of its own, choosing a 'seated sport' like cycling as your main mode of exercise adds to them if 'corrective' or 'balancing' exercises aren't incorporated into your health and fitness plan.

The primal patterns and their importance to cyclists

The human body is an amazingly versatile movement machine. Alongside 'gait', all other human movements can be broken down into combinations of squatting, lunging, bending, pushing, pulling and twisting.

In his book *How to Eat, Move and Be Healthy!*, Paul Chek explains the significance of these 'primal pattern movements' like this:

If you couldn't correctly perform these seven movement patterns quickly and effectively without thinking about what your body was doing, you probably wouldn't survive in the wild. Even though our lifestyle is very different from our developmental ancestors, these seven movement patterns are still key to performing daily tasks and staying injury free. (Chek, 2004)

Many sports still rely on these movement patterns in developing the athletes' ability to play the game. Rugby players, for example, who run, throw and tackle as part of their training, incorporate many of the primal patterns as part of their conditioning. A sport like rugby allows the human body to maintain the kind of physical conditioning that would have been part of our daily lives as more primitive human beings. The human athlete is on his/her feet, moving in short bursts in multiple directions, generating force from the ground up to throw, tackle, push and pull.

In general, we are designed for short bursts of strength-based activity interspersed with light activity or rest. In terms of 'primal endurance', walking or jogging would have been the main mode of movement, with long-distance endurance running becoming useful and specialized in certain circumstances.

Functional strength basics for cyclists

The word 'functional' is used widely in health and fitness to describe an ability to perform daily tasks effectively and problem free. In a sporting context it is also used to describe your ability to carry out the athletic demands of the sport.

In this book, the 'primal patterns' form the functional foundation that will keep you pain and injury free and help you excel as a cyclist. In practical terms you will see them in Chapter 3, illustrating essential strength exercises for cyclists.

Although modern lifestyles are fairly sedentary, lifting, carrying and moving objects are still common movements that everyone will encounter and need to manage in order to avoid injury. Sports people engaged in activities that require strength as part of the game will be aware of their strength and conditioning status by way of their performance. To continue the rugby analogy, most players will be lifting and moving weights in the gym in addition to their sport-specific drills on the field to facilitate better performance. Most people (including cyclists) who are not engaged in fitness training of this type will only become aware of their lack of conditioning when they become injured, often when they have to lift, move or carry something heavy unexpectedly.

Many sports like rugby have inherent 'functional strength' elements included in them, but endurance sports like cycling are highly repetitive and relatively 'low load', negating the core stimulus of ground forces while developing the cardiovascular system or 'engine' in relative isolation.

Lots of people who love cycling are not naturally 'sporty' types. They often report that they were not good at sports at school because they lacked the natural strength, coordination and speed required for more 'functional' sports like rugby or hockey. They may have started to ride a bike later in life to commute to work, and then almost accidentally found themselves riding further and faster and enjoying cycling as a sport and pastime in itself.

Even those who consider themselves 'endurance athletes' will often have specialized quite early to the detriment of developing more varied movement abilities and motor programmes, and will therefore be disadvantaged in terms of strength. For example, like many others I know, I went from being a competitive swimmer to being a competitive cyclist, and aside from the few hours of more general PE at school, my feet never really touched the ground.

General conditioning vs cycling specific training

Several physiological and theoretical arguments have held cyclists back from pursuing conditioning exercise off the bike as part of their training.

At its extreme, the 'sport-specific training' proposition suggests that any time spent on more 'general' conditioning activities takes up valuable cycling time and represents a distraction at best and a detrimental influence at worse.

The main thrust of this theoretical and practical approach is supported by established sports science, which proves that performance on the bike is largely determined by the physiology of your cardiovascular system or aerobic 'engine', and therefore the bulk of training should be spent targeting these elements through the cycling movements themselves. This allows for maximal adaptation of not only the central cardiovascular systems of the heart and lungs, but also all the peripheral changes that occur at the muscular and cellular levels as you pedal.

In light of this physiological understanding, strength training could be considered counterproductive for several reasons. Firstly, since strength is not a primary determinant of cycling performance, there seems little benefit to be gained from time spent on it, especially for 'amateur' cyclists for whom time is precious.

Secondly, there is the fear that strength training will result in muscle development and bulk that will diminish performance by way of making the cyclist heavier. In a sport where your 'power to weight' ratio is highly relevant when you point your bike uphill, there is real legitimacy to this reasoning.

Finally, even when considering the strength elements of cycling that are notable for all cyclists, such as seated and standing climbing and sprinting, there is the argument that off-the-bike conditioning is not specific enough, because the movements involved (such as pushing, pulling and squatting) do not have any direct 'carry over' to cycling.

In this book I will show you that most of the benefits of the 'primal pattern' strength training (together with corrective stretching and core work) are indirect. That is to say, they benefit the cyclist by way of maintaining human 'norms' that prevent injury both on and off the bike rather than directly improving cycling fitness. These indirect benefits include better health, greater consistency and robustness in training, and a more linear progression.

Having said that, I fully understand the need for specialization in training to become a 'cyclist', and I am not suggesting that 'general conditioning' becomes the main focus of any cyclist's training programme. However, I am suggesting that this overspecialization can lead to problems that can easily be prevented with a little time spent on off-the-bike essentials. This is where a corrective or balancing approach comes into its own, by introducing the essential conditioning that will keep you functionally fit both on and off the bike, in the minimum time.

Essentials of on- and off-the-bike training

In recognizing the physiological importance of sport-specific training, to consider yourself a 'cyclist' most of your training time should be spent on the bike, refining your cycling-specific aerobic fitness and movement patterns. For this reason, I would suggest that two-thirds to three-quarters of the time you spend exercising per week should be spent on the bike. The remaining quarter to a third should be spent on conditioning work, focused on improving those elements that you lack the most.

Cycling movements are very different from those that I am about to introduce, and there are some specific strength requirements that must be developed on the bike itself, where you are pushing harder on the flats, climbing in and out of the saddle, or sprinting as hard as you can. I want to make it clear that these elements are essential to achieving your peak potential as a cyclist, and become particularly important in semi-competitive or competitive situations. The off-the-bike essential conditioning in this book provides the foundation for the sport-specific strength and skill that must then be developed on the bike to maximize your potential gains.

On-the-bike strengthening techniques and practices are outside the scope of this book, but are an essential part of an optimal training programme. I will hint at where these elements fit in throughout Chapter 6 on periodization and planning.

For now, I want to introduce each of the primal patterns since they are so important and provide a framework for the biological norms or standards we should all be aiming for. I will illustrate in brief some of the day-to-day activities that require these movements, and highlight the problems and injuries that might develop from deconditioning. Later, in the essential strength section of Chapter 3, I will show you how to train them yourself.

Squatting

Squatting is essentially any sitting movement.

In day-to-day situations, its most common use would be in combination with a bend to lift an object off the ground and move it forwards or overhead. It is important to maintain an inwards curve of the lower back. This approach to lifting/moving weight is also referred to as a 'neutral spine philosophy' and will be discussed further in the strength section of Chapter 3.

In terms of 'sport-specific' carry-over, the squat forms the foundation for standing/ sprinting power on the bike, as it is the foundational movement for any 'jump'. Squat work can be dovetailed with cycling-specific accelerations or 'jumps' to translate gains in strength to speed and power on the bike, particularly for accelerations out of the saddle, either on the flat or uphill.

Bending

A relaxed bend posture relies on the passive flexibility of the 'posterior chain' of muscles and tissues to reach the ground, while saving energy in the muscles of the legs. If you can't touch the ground with straight legs you have lost some of your flexibility in the bend.

Flexion dominance is a term used to describe the movement bias in most people's daily lives towards forwards bending or flexion. Where backwards bending (or extension) is not part of our daily vocabulary, problems can develop because we can become unbalanced.

A bending movement is one that allows us to pick objects off the ground or below us, or reach for something by leaning forwards.

Under light loads a straight-legged bend saves energy in the leg muscles and relies on the elasticity of the fascia (connective tissue) along the back of the body.

Lifting/moving a heavier load off the ground requires a different bend movement, using slightly bent legs to recruit the hip muscles (buttocks) to support and share the load with the back, and working with the lumbar spine as 'neutral' as possible.

To distinguish between the squat and bend, in a squat the load is above your centre of gravity, while in a bend it is below. In the squat a knee bend initiates the movement and the torso stays relatively upright, while in the bend a tipping at the hips/back initiates the movement and the knees bend as a secondary motion.

Range of movement in bending is often inhibited by shortened hamstring muscles at the back of the thigh, a common consequence of sedentary lifestyles and a lot of time spent sitting in chairs. A bend combined with a twist is the most common movement that injures the lower back due to lack of conditioning, for example by lifting things awkwardly off the floor or out of a car.

For cyclists who experience lower back ache with riding of any kind, or even worse experience the onset of neurological symptoms (weakness or shooting pains) when riding, a close look at deficits in flexibility or strength in the 'bend' pattern is critical.

Of all the 'primal patterns', I would say a deficit in your ability to bend is most likely to cause injury and diminish your performance on the bike. A deficit may be anywhere along the spectrum of flexibility, core stability and strength, or most likely a combination of all three interrelated elements. This is why you will see many exercises in this book that 'correct' for this most common dysfunction by way of both strengthening the back in a backwards bend and also lengthening the hamstrings.

Lunging

Lunging movements are those involving a step or stride with one foot in front of the other where both legs bend and one foot leaves the ground.

A lunge is less stable than a squat or bend, but more versatile when linking other movements and is common in many sports and games that require a rapid change of direction when running around the field or court.

A lunge often connects force between the legs and upper body through the core when combined with a twist, transmitting force from the ground up, and expressing it through the torso and arms. In conditioning terms, the 'typical' lunge is forwards, but a lunge can be multidirectional too, moving the body or force backwards or sideways or somewhere in between.

A 'split squat' is a more controlled, less dynamic version of the same movement, where both feet stay on the ground and the torso moves up and down. A split squat can be used to create more balanced strength in the movement before adding power and pace in the more dynamic 'sporting' lunge.

Lunging before you have a good grounding in a 'split squat' can be aggravating for those not used to the deceleration forces involved, or for those with a 'quad dominant' muscle imbalance pattern. Cyclists often fall into this category, and so for these reasons I have chosen to include the split squat rather than the lunge in Chapter 3 on essential strength exercises for cyclists.

The split squat is a great addition to any cyclist's conditioning programme as it is more challenging in the frontal and transverse planes (at the sides and in rotation) than the more symmetrical movements of the bend and squat, and therefore helps to promote multiplanar stability when practised with good form. Also in a split stance

any asymmetries in leg, hip and core strength and alignment can be more easily identified and addressed.

If you are a cyclist who doesn't have a background in running or games it may be safest to strengthen your split squat technique first, before lunging, or before introducing any games or multidirectional sports as part of your cross-training. Selecting and integrating appropriate cross-training elements to suit you will be discussed further in Chapter 6.

Pushing

A pushing movement is one where you exert force to move something away from you, or move yourself away from a solid surface such as a wall or the ground.

In any standing push in the functional or primal sense, force is generated from the ground up via the legs and transmitted through the core or trunk to be expressed through the chest and arms.

Pushing movements may be single arm or double arm, with single-arm movements often being combined with a twist through the upper body and a counterrotation on the opposite side. Punching or throwing actions are good examples of explosive single-arm 'push' movements.

Double-arm pushes can exert more force (but not necessarily speed), and for all-round conditioning it is important to train both single- and double-arm variations. A common fault with a push is to excessively round the upper back through the movement and thrust the head forwards of the body. This is particularly common for people with poor posture who are stiff and slumped through the upper back and tight in the chest, a posture common in cyclists who sit at a desk for most of their day.

Although there is not much direct carry-over with pushing movements on the bike, as part of maintaining a balanced conditioning programme functional pushes are important. For this reason, standing pushing exercises should be your first choice since they have the most practical carry-over to real-life situations. More isolated pushes can be used to develop the abdominals or to balance or correct for core weakness. A push-up is an example of a relatively isolated core exercise that is often used in this way to strengthen the core.

Pulling

A pulling movement is one where you exert force to move something towards you, or move yourself closer to a solid object.

Functional pulling movements are performed standing up with force generated from the ground up through the legs and core and expressed through the arms. The exception is in 'pull-up' or climbing movements, where force is generated by the back and arms with a co-contraction of the core/trunk musculature.

Pulling movements may be single arm or double arm, with single-arm movements often being combined with a twist through the upper body and a counterrotation on the opposite side.

The main conditioning exercises for developing pulling strength are variations of rowing movements, which develop the large 'lat' muscles that give a triangular shape to the back of the body from the shoulders to the waist, the rhomboids between the shoulder blades, as well as the biceps at the front of the arms. The row can be performed in relative isolation first, to develop upper back strength and then integrated with other patterns for a more 'functional' movement in the true sense.

Isolated exercises are those that target specific muscles or areas of muscles that have become weak or need development. **Integrated exercises** work the whole body, relying on chains or 'teams' of muscles working together to generate strength and power. In this book there are relatively isolated strength exercises for the back and abdominal muscles in the core section of Chapter 4, to target the areas that often become weak in cyclists. The exercises in the strength section of Chapter 3 are relatively integrated, to teach the body to move as a working whole. In practice it is often wise to isolate first, then integrate, which is why for many readers it would be sensible to work on the stretching and core essentials first (in Chapters 2 and 4), before introducing the strength exercises (in Chapter 3).

Isolated exercises for the back (such as the prone cobra in the Core section of this book) help correct for the cycling posture, which tends to stretch and weaken the mid and lower back musculature. These movements are often necessary as an adjunct to the main movements where the muscles are particularly weak. Ideally, more integrated pulling movements (such as the bent-over row in the essential strength section) should be included too. If you have access to a cable machine in a gym, this is one of the best 'free weight' tools to finally assimilate pulling movements with lunges, squats, bends and twists to improve the carry-over to standing strength on the bike.

Pulling movements should be a priority in any cyclist's training programme because of their postural benefits both on and off the bike. They can also improve performance when a rider stands out of the saddle and pulls on the bars in coordination with the drive generated by the legs.

Twisting

Twisting movements are some of the most important of all the primal movement patterns as they connect, link and facilitate so many of the others.

Force generated from the ground is transferred through the core via a twist in any single-arm asymmetrical movement, such as the pulls and pushes described on the preceding pages. In almost all 'functional' movements, the feet are anchored and the torso or trunk rotates above the pelvis, transferring load and speed through the core to the arms.

In many real-life lifting situations a bend is combined with a twist, since often the object we are trying to pick up off the floor cannot be approached symmetrically or 'square on'. This combination of bending and twisting is the movement with which many people (including cyclists) injure their lower back, giving good reason to ensure conditioning in both movements separately, as well as combining them.

The root causes of bend and twist injuries are often a combination of lack of flexibility in the hamstrings, lack of abdominal engagement on a forward bend, and poor movement technique between the back and the legs in the coordination of the movement itself. This provocative combination can injure cyclists, keeping them off the bike for an extended period.

In conditioning terms, the classic integrated (functional and on your feet) twisting movements are variations of the 'chop', in which the prime movers are the abdominal obliques that rotate the torso, together with the associated 'anterior sling' muscles from the adductor of the inner thigh to the opposite shoulder. In the 'reverse chop' (its opposing movement) the prime movers are those that rotate the core from behind – the 'posterior sling' from the glute of the grounded leg to the opposite latissimus dorsi (Chek, 2004). In more isolated examples, many crawling and crunching variations involve an opposing leg and arm action and target the twist movement for a functional core.

Including twisting exercises as part of your programme is important to maintain the mobility of your spine in particular. Isolated twists can also be a good way to strengthen your abdominal muscles without becoming flexion dominant by way of too many 'crunch' type exercises.

Gait – walking and running

Walking and running are undoubtedly our most basic of human movements. Our upright posture and our ability to move easily and efficiently on two feet are at the heart of our movement potential.

Remembering and reminding our bodies how to walk and run with good posture and alignment can help us maintain our musculoskeletal health and well-being, and enables us to participate in many complementary sports and activities.

You would think that walking at the very least was something we all do every day, and for the most part that's true. But consciously walking or running for health and well-being in a mindful way, rather than rushing around carrying heavy bags or running for a train, can be an important part of a balanced conditioning programme. For some, cycling is an attractive option because of pain and injury issues associated with running or running sports. But even for those who have turned to cycling for its low-impact cardiovascular benefits, maintaining a minimal amount of walking to keep the joints and bones healthy should be an essential.

Knowing where to start

Understanding human movement and the importance of functional strength is one thing, but knowing where to start on your own conditioning programme can be something else altogether. In my experience, with all the best intentions in the world 'paralysis by analysis' is one of the biggest barriers to actually getting stuck into some exercise that might change your body for the better. Fear of 'doing it wrong' is one of the main reasons cyclists fail to start on a conditioning programme, but in this book I'm going to make it as easy as possible for you to do something practical straight away.

Following the 'success formula'

Cyclists are often put off conditioning exercises because even if they believe them to be beneficial in theory, in practice they are concerned about causing injury or excessive muscle soreness that will have an immediate and undesirable impact on their cycling. The reason for this is simple.

For many cyclists, to launch in with whole-body strengthening exercises represents a challenge above their current level of overall condition. Just because you are a fit cyclist on the bike does not mean that you are a fit human being off it.

You may have a developed cardiovascular system, but that does not make you any more able to move well off the bike, or any less likely to injure yourself by accident lifting weights or even moving your own body weight in an unusual way. The truth is that in the broader sense you may be relatively out of shape, so it's hardly surprising that the sudden introduction of dynamic conditioning work can be uncomfortable, and in some cases risky.

Muscle soreness is one of the main reasons cyclists avoid other exercise, and this unfamiliar 'symptom' discourages riders from taking their off-the-bike training any further than the first troublesome experiments. When something that is supposed to be beneficial makes cycling uncomfortable or more difficult, as a rider you are fairly quickly persuaded away from the arguments altogether. However, if you choose the exercises that are most appropriate to you by using the examples in this book, you will experience minimal soreness and maximal gains. If you overstretch a muscle, or work too hard on a strength exercise, you will notice some muscle soreness, granted, but in this book I am encouraging you to exercise little and often so that your immediate impressions are that you feel better, on and off the bike, not worse.

The key to harnessing the benefits of *Ride Strong: Essential Conditioning for Cyclists* is to select exercises that are at the right level for you and respect the 'success formula'. The success formula states that the more deconditioned you are, the more likely you will need to focus on exercises to the left of the equation, and then progressively shift your emphasis steadily towards the right (so flexibility first, then core stability and then strength).

Through years of working one to one with clients and with the application of the principles I have learned through my studies with the CHEK institute, I have found this success formula concept is key to choosing exercises that are right for you. I hope that through the course of this book you too can grasp the basics that will inform your exercise choices.

 # The success formula

Remember the
success formula:

FLEXIBILITY
+ CORE STABILITY
+ STRENGTH
= POWER POTENTIAL

Both new and experienced cyclists may neglect the need for all-round conditioning, and some may never have strengthened their body through the essential primal patterns that will be outlined in their basic form in Chapter 3. If this describes you, or you turned to cycling because of injury problems in another sport, start by balancing the muscles in your body first by stretching, and improving your core stability and control, before finally moving on to the strength basics outlined in this book.

I have structured this book so that as your physical condition improves, you can progressively add exercises in the correct order through the different stages as outlined in Chapter 6.

If you have not done any 'conditioning' exercise for a while, designing a programme that includes just stretching and core essentials may be the best way to start. Just skip the 'Strength' part altogether in Chapter 3 to start with.

If you find that in working through the stretching essentials you are extremely tight, then a stretch-only programme may be even better.

If you don't use it you lose it – and how to get it back

Flexibility first

When the neuromuscular systems are understimulated they tend to lose their inherent memory and muscle balance. Muscles that are not regularly stretched become short and tight, and those that are not worked become weak. A nervous system that once had a memory for a movement like a squat may lose track of that memory, or find it altered or changed to work around restrictions and tightness.

When you come from a place of relative deconditioning, you have to re-establish normal length-tension relationships in muscles and around joints as a priority before reintroducing whole body strength movements. This is why re-establishing flexibility and mobility norms with the essential stretches for cyclists in Chapter 2 should be the first priority.

Core isolation second

Where one muscle has become short or tight, another corresponding muscle often begins to weaken. Sometimes the weakness happens first due to lack of stimulus through ground forces or loading, and then the body tends to tighten up in an attempt to stabilize. Either way, together with improving and restoring flexibility, re-establishing core control and stability in the trunk should be the next priority.

Pre-stretching the short and tight muscles before strengthening the weak areas in relative isolation is the key to changing the body, moving it towards better balance and optimal performance on the bike.

The essential core exercises in Chapter 4 will help you identify and isolate key weak spots to that you can re-establish good posture, control and muscle balance. For most readers, I would recommend designing a programme from the essential stretches (Chapter 2) and essential core exercises (Chapter 4) to start with.

Integrated strength last

The essential strength exercises for cyclists in Chapter 3 represent a reintroduction of the more integrated primal patterns that I have explained here. Some of you will be able to incorporate these straight away, or as part of a periodized plan during your 'off season', whereas others will do better to focus on the stretching and core exercise for a little longer.

If you have not done any off-the-bike conditioning before or for some time, I recommend you leave out Chapter 3 for your first year of conditioning. Equally, if you start your essential exercise plan during the season when you are doing the most riding, you may want to save the introduction of the strength exercise for your off season.

Once you are confident with the core exercises, and/or you are in your off season, I recommend you introduce the essential strength exercises for cyclists in Chapter 3 of this book. I have explained the essential exercises in Chapters 2, 3 and 4 in the order of stretch, strength and core, as this is the order in which you would write them into a programme that includes all three elements. The details of how to choose your exercises within a seasonal plan are outlined in Chapter 6 of this book on programme design and periodization.

The emphasis of your programme should change according to the season, as well as in respect of your physical condition when you start your plan. The exercises you are using within your programme should vary and change at least every 8–12 weeks to keep your body adapting and developing by way of a change of stimulus. The essential exercises in this book, together with the recommendations regarding cross-training in Chapter 5, should be all you need as a time-squeezed cyclist to ride strong all year round.

2. Essential stretches

Overview of this chapter

- **Mobilizations and stretches for the hips and legs** (page 63)
  - » Piriformis stretch
  - » Wall glute stretch (post-exercise only)
  - » Iliotibial band (ITB) foam roller mobilization
  - » Swiss ball quad and hip flexor stretch
  - » The hamstrings stretches
  - » Supine knee extension
  - » Supine knee extension – strap assisted
  - » Active isolated stretching (AIS) style – strap assisted
  - » Passive doorframe stretch – post-exercise only
- **Stretches for neck and upper back** (page 83)
  - » Upper trapezius neck stretch
  - » Sternocleidomastoid (SCM) neck stretch

ESSENTIAL STRETCHES READY REFERENCE PICTURES (page 89)

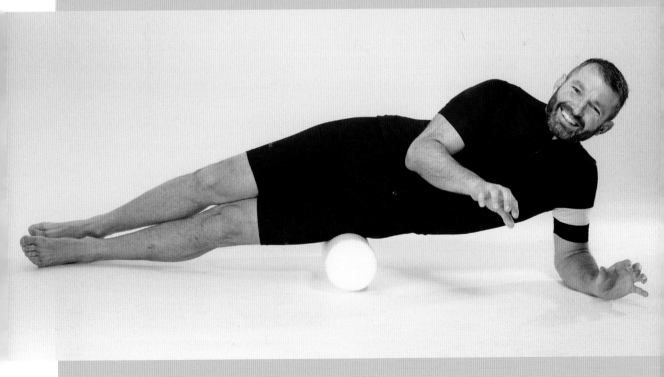

Why should cyclists stretch?

There has been a lot of confusion about whether stretching is beneficial for cyclists and which stretches are the most suitable, as well as how and when to stretch to maximize the performance benefits and minimize the risk of injury. There are many reasons why you might stretch and each kind of stretching requires a different approach depending on its goal.

The approach I am taking in this book is to illustrate some essential stretches that will help prevent progressive tightness and stiffness in areas that can become a tendency in cyclists. When cyclists get stiff and tight, injury issues can develop and performance can be limited. The goal of the stretches in this book is to restore and maintain normal mobility and length-tension relationships in the muscles and joints to maximize cycling performance and reduce risk of injury.

The stretches are designed to balance the tightening and immobility that can result from hours spent on the bike, as well as for cycling muscles that can tend to shorten. They also take into account the fact that many cyclists are also office workers, who sit at a desk for most of the day.

Many forms of exercise incorporate elements of flexibility work, but if you are chronically stiff in specific areas, the easiest way to have a tangible impact on your flexibility is to tackle each area one at a time, with isolated, targeted stretches.

The cross-training options that might enhance your flexibility further if you find that you are stiff will be discussed later in Chapter 5, but the best way to have an impact is using the isolated stretches here.

Combination stretches that stretch multiple chains of muscles can miss the target area, and the stiffer you are the harder it is to get these more complex positions right. Where muscles in a chain are short and tight, there may be no impact on muscle balance as a whole, and at worst the 'longer' muscles may lengthen further, exacerbating the imbalance and leading to a worsening of symptoms and poorer performance.

For example, many commonly performed hamstring stretches are combination stretches for the hamstrings at the knee and hip, together with the lower back. A typical example might be the 'toe touch' stretch from standing. Cyclists need to be more specific in targeting the lower hamstrings at the knee to have a big impact: the 'supine' stretches where you lie on your back and raise your leg are usually a better choice. This is why all the hamstring stretches included in this chapter are performed from a supine position.

In practice, learning to extend or arch the lower back throughout the hamstring stretch is the key to hitting the area behind the knee. This technique can be difficult to start with and requires practice maintaining this lumbar curve. Later in this chapter there will be four examples of hamstring stretches that will hit the tightest parts of the muscle group without overstretching the lower back.

The essential stretches in this chapter target one muscle or specific area at a time in a focused way. These focused isolations should form the foundation of your stretching programme until you find that you are flexible in all the areas we are working through here.

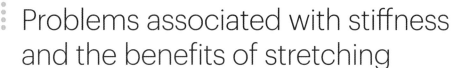

Problems associated with stiffness and the benefits of stretching

Feeling stiff and tight is quite common, but don't presume that this is 'normal' or something you just need to accept and get used to as a cyclist. In fact you might not even be aware that you have symptoms of tightness, so here are some clues that you may need to work on your flexibility, and some of the benefits you should expect from consistent, intelligent stretching.

Symptoms of stiffness and tightness

- Discomfort and a feeling of inflexibility
- Muscle cramping on and off the bike
- Muscle injury on and off the bike (strains)
- Joint and connective tissue injuries (sprains)
- Joint degeneration (in the spine, knees and neck in particular)
- Poor posture off the bike
- Poor bike fit (posture on the bike) and power associated with limited range of movement

Benefits associated with stretching

- An improved feeling of body 'balance' on and off the bike
- Reduced risk of injury of any kind on and off the bike
- Improved potential for optimal bike fit
- Improved power and pedalling efficiency as a result
- Improved posture and performance on and off the bike

If you find the stretches in this section relatively easy to perform or feel little real 'stretch' in the more flexible examples given, you may be better off going straight to the essential strength and core sections of this book in Chapters 3 and 4. For some of the female readership in particular this may be the case as I have found women to be generally more flexible than men.

The more difficult you find the stretches in this section, the more you should persist with them until you improve, and the more emphasis you should place on stretching in your overall programme.

The success formula dictates that you prioritize each stage progressively in order to maximize your progress, so if you are very stiff you will do well to focus on these essential stretches before introducing some core stability exercises from Chapter 4. Only then would you move on to the more integrated strength elements in Chapter 3 of this book.

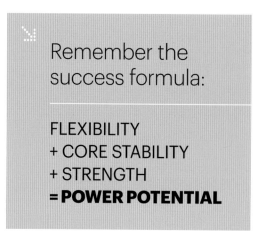

Remember the success formula:

FLEXIBILITY
+ CORE STABILITY
+ STRENGTH
= **POWER POTENTIAL**

Positional problem areas for cyclists

Some of the stiffness and tightness associated with cycling is a result of the cycling position, or baseline 'posture'. In addition, the repetitive movements of the cycling action cause some classically short and tight areas too, and it is these two elements – the fundamental position and the repetitive movements – that can lead to tightness.

Any posture is the position from which movement begins and ends, and for cyclists the bike position can contribute to problems if no balancing movements are included in a conditioning programme. Some of the essential mobilizations and stretches in this section focus on restoring the normal range of motion in the muscles and joints that is restricted or limited by the cycling position.

As human beings we have a 'physiological norm' for movement, which is our standing posture. This is the position we are biomechanically designed to move from and to, and so the seated position we move from on a bicycle represents a significant deviation that can lead to issues developing, reducing our movement potential or efficiency.

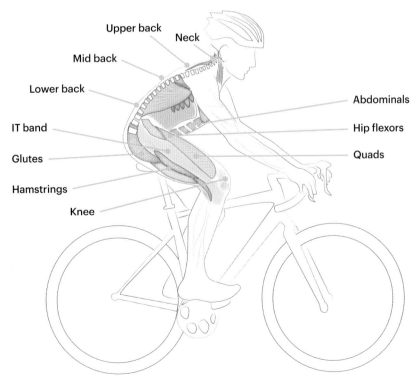

Upper back
Neck
Mid back
Lower back
Abdominals
IT band
Hip flexors
Glutes
Quads
Hamstrings
Knee

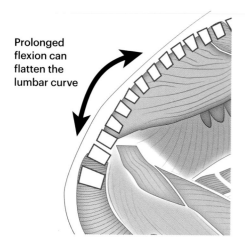

Prolonged flexion can flatten the lumbar curve

The cyclist's spine

Lower back (lumbar spine)

Seated in the saddle, the lower back suffers from prolonged flexion and flattening. Stiffness is the least of the problems that can start here, and because the alignment of the lower back is the furthest from its physiological upright 'norm' when cycling, it is often the area that cyclists are aware of the most. Ensuring that your 'bike fit' is balanced can reduce the postural stress in this area, but over time, even on a well-balanced bike, this relatively 'unnatural' position can take its toll.

As the lumbar spine becomes progressively flattened from riding (and sitting), the lower back muscles tend to weaken. A weak back (and core) will ache even more when standing or climbing for long periods, leading to fatigue, instability and loss of power.

Over time, where the lumbar spine has become flattened the lumbar discs can begin to migrate backwards, which together with weakened abdominal muscles leads to a dull ache across the lower back and sometimes weakness or referred pain down one or both legs. At worst, a disc 'bulge' or injury can occur when lifting or moving suddenly, particularly when bending forwards. These back issues can often become quite serious and lead to long periods of rehabilitation and treatment, meaning enforced time spent off the bike.

A disc 'bulge' is a common term for a more properly named disc herniation. Cyclists are at an increased risk of this kind of injury in the lower back because of their postural tendencies and lack of conditioning in lifting and carrying movements. If you imagine the discs of your lower back as being like Jaffa cakes with a soft supportive jelly centre, a disc 'bulge' occurs when the jelly centre is squeezed backwards or to one side and begins to push out into the space where the nerves run along the spine and out to the limbs. This unexpected obstruction can cause pain in the lower back and sometimes (when the bulge is sideways) into the hips and legs. Disc injuries at their worst can have a long-term impact on your ability to ride a bike pain free. Maintaining normal curves in the spine, good length in the hamstrings and a functional core when lifting can prevent these problems from developing.

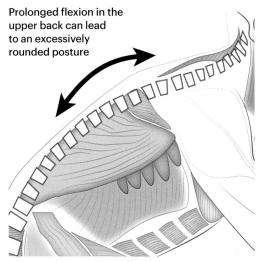

Prolonged flexion in the upper back can lead to an excessively rounded posture

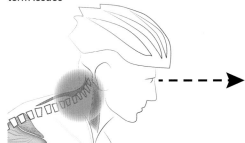

The stiffer the upper back, the more extension is needed in the neck to look forwards at the road ahead. Prolonged stress in this area can lead to bony changes in the neck, and longer term issues

Upper back (thoracic spine)

The mid back between the shoulder blades also suffers from prolonged immobility on the bike. Normally moving and rotating when walking or running, when seated on a bike the thoracic spine becomes a stationary bridge connecting the upper body with the driving force of the legs and hips.

This can result in poor posture in the upper back as the spine becomes 'fixed' and 'rounded', even when the cyclist stands upright. This poor posture can also lead to knock-on shoulder problems, most often experienced off the bike in situations where you reach or carry loads overhead.

Neck (cervical spine)

Naturally the eyes need to be looking to the horizon if you want to see where you are going, as well as what's coming. Coupled with the forwards bend through the upper back to reach the bars, the neck curves inwards to look forwards at the road ahead. Often the neck can cope well with this extension provided the rest of the spine is moving well, but if the spine becomes stiff lower down there can be excessive load 'referred' up towards the neck that can lead to more serious problems.

Where there is prolonged postural stress at the junction between the upper back and neck, the bones of the spine can change shape as the body attempts to stabilize the area. This can lead to arthritic symptoms such as pain in the neck and down the arms, as well as occasional headaches and dizziness when looking up. Although these changes take many years to develop, they can be prevented with a proactive approach to mobilizing the spine and stretching the muscles around the shoulders and neck.

My essential mobilizations for the spine focus on extension (backwards bending) of the lumbar spine (lower back), rotation and extension of the thoracic spine (upper back), and flexion (forwards bending) of the cervical spine (neck). These movements need to be emphasized by cyclists who spend unnatural amounts of time in a flexed position.

'Flexion dominance' is a term used to describe the tendency of many people (cyclists included) to have many more forward-bending (flexion, picture left) movements in their day-to-day lives than backward-bending (extension, picture right) ones. Lack of extension in your movement vocabulary can cause problems, so introducing some extension exercises can help to balance the body.

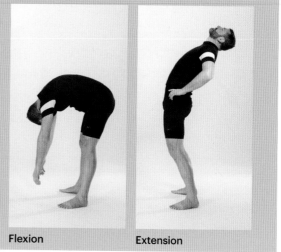

Flexion   Extension

Muscles of the upper body and neck

Although not a prime mover when seated in the saddle, the upper body can get tight and tense through resting a fair amount of your body weight on the handlebars as you ride. Holding the bars for prolonged periods can create tension and postural load up the arms to the upper back and neck. Consequently, even when practising good form by keeping the elbows bent and the arms somewhat 'active', the muscles of the chest and upper back can get short and tight.

Over time, 'trigger points' can develop in the upper trapezius muscles of the upper back in particular, which will be felt as hard, uncomfortable 'knots' in the muscle that can cause pain. While stretching the chest can be achieved to some degree as you mobilize the spine, the neck and upper back muscles can be more difficult to effectively stretch in some cases without the addition of deep tissue massage.

'Trigger points' are so called because they can be felt as a localized 'lump' of muscle or tissue that is at the centre of, or the source of, discomfort or pain in a muscle. The discomfort or pain may be on the spot itself, or may radiate out from the trouble spot when it is pressed or irritated. 'Trigger point therapy' is a term given to treatment of these trouble spots either by a therapist or by self-massage techniques and tools.

My essential stretches for the muscles of the upper body and neck focus on the areas that tighten from holding the handlebars for prolonged periods. If you regularly suffer from neck discomfort, including some remedial or 'sports' massage as part of your training plan, together with the stretches here, will maximize your progress.

Tightness caused by the cycling action

As well as mobilizing and stretching areas that get tight because of the cycling position, the working muscles will need regular stretching too to enhance and improve recovery between sessions.

My essential stretches for the hip and leg muscles focus on the areas that work the hardest or within a shortened range at various stages in the cycling pedal stroke. Isolating these specific areas is important for you to avoid muscle imbalances developing that lead to inefficiencies and increased risk of injury.

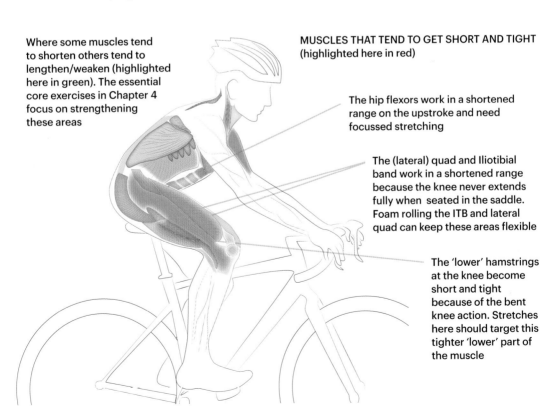

Where some muscles tend to shorten others tend to lengthen/weaken (highlighted here in green). The essential core exercises in Chapter 4 focus on strengthening these areas

MUSCLES THAT TEND TO GET SHORT AND TIGHT (highlighted here in red)

The hip flexors work in a shortened range on the upstroke and need focussed stretching

The (lateral) quad and Iliotibial band work in a shortened range because the knee never extends fully when seated in the saddle. Foam rolling the ITB and lateral quad can keep these areas flexible

The 'lower' hamstrings at the knee become short and tight because of the bent knee action. Stretches here should target this tighter 'lower' part of the muscle

While the quadriceps (at the front of the thigh) is one of the prime movers for cyclists, one of the worst problem areas for tightness is often the hamstrings at the back of the knee. Though the hamstrings assist in the downstroke at the hip, and are prime movers in the upstroke at the knee, they are far less dominant at most intensities than the quads. At moderate intensities the downstroke is the major contributor to power production on flat roads. The upstroke only really becomes a major player when the ground goes up, or when you start to really go hard. However, because the knees rarely straighten completely (except for when a cyclist stands out of the saddle), the hamstrings can be one of the most problematic areas for cyclists, and even more so for those who sit at a desk for work. Stretching the hamstrings effectively is therefore very important for cyclists, even though as a muscle group they do not contribute to the action as much as the quads.

Of the quads at the front of the thigh, the lateral portion (the outer thigh) can become dominant and tight together with the iliotibial band (ITB) of connective tissue that runs from the outer hip to the outside of the knee joint. This 'fascia' has a poor blood supply and is made of tougher stuff than muscles, and therefore responds best to self-massage techniques together with stretches that target the tightest parts of the quads.

'Fascia' is the term given to a band of connective tissue that attaches, stabilizes, encloses and connects muscles or organs of the body. Collectively these fascial layers form a complex, layered web of tissue throughout the whole body. Maintaining the pliability of these tissues is as important as maintaining muscle length. 'Myofascial' is a collective term given to a muscle and the connective tissue surrounding and relating to it. Foam rolling the lateral thigh can be called a myofascial release technique because it impacts both the iliotibial band and lateral quadriceps muscle.

Throughout this chapter I refer to 'upper' and 'lower' or 'inner' and 'outer' portions of muscle groups. This is in reference to how the muscles work during the cycling action or to which area is the tightest or weakest. Anatomically, there is no upper or lower hamstring, for example, but in describing the different parts in this way I hope to help you understand their function and target each exercise more effectively to the most relevant part of the muscle.

The Essential Stretches

Mobilizations and stretches for the spine and back

Before stretching any muscles around the back it's important to mobilize the joints and structures of the spine itself. Stretches for the back muscles can be helpful, but direct and specific mobilizations for the vertebrae of the spine are also needed in order to keep each segment moving and to avoid the stiffness and rigidity developing.

With 24 bones or 'vertebrae' in the spine, there are a lot of joints to consider and where stiffness develops in any one joint, the movement of the joints above and below will be affected and tightness in the surrounding muscles is likely to follow. The spine really is the 'deep core' of your body, not only providing it with physical structure, but also protecting the spinal cord that runs through the vertebrae. All movement is *neuro*muscular, and maintaining a healthy support structure for your nervous system as well as your muscles is absolutely critical in achieving and maintaining your physical potential.

Between each vertebra is a supportive cartilaginous 'disc' that allows for some movement but also cushions against load, particularly in the lumbar spine, which is designed to support the most weight. Healthy discs maintain a healthy nervous system by ensuring enough space between the joints, which in turn allows room for the nerves to exit the spine to the limbs.

Ligaments run the length of the spine too, bridging all the vertebrae and linking the bones together, and

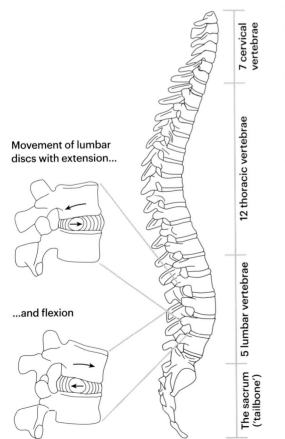

Movement of lumbar discs with extension...

...and flexion

7 cervical vertebrae

12 thoracic vertebrae

5 lumbar vertebrae

The sacrum ('tailbone')

these need to be stretched and maintained to stay healthy and flexible. If these ligaments become less pliable and more rigid they can buckle and begin to encroach on the space where the nerves need to 'run'.

As a functional whole, maintaining the structural integrity of the spine in terms of its postural curves and movement potential is essential to avoid any irreversible degenerative changes to the bones, discs or ligaments that can limit your cycling performance. Maintaining range of movement in the joints and keeping muscles flexible is also the first step in maintaining good posture. Establishing core control and normal movement patterns are the second and third key elements.

Mobilizations for the thoracic spine (upper back)

The lower back is a known problem area for many cyclists, but the upper back, or thoracic spine, deserves just as much if not more attention. Spending hours hunched over the handlebars and often crouched over a desk too can lead to stiffness in the upper back and significant issues around your neck and shoulders. The stiffer your upper back, the more likely you are to develop a sore neck.

While the lower back needs some attention, first mobilizing the thoracic spine in rotation and then extension can help maximize the benefits of the stretches and mobilizations for the lower back that follow. Completing the stretches and mobilizations in the order in which they appear in this essential stretches section will give you the greatest benefits.

Designed in particular for rotation, the thoracic vertebrae can get 'stuck' when you spend a lot of time flexed forward, and this can restrict twisting and backwards bending. Contrary to what seems logical, this also limits how well you bend forwards, thereby having a direct impact on your cycling position and your ability to achieve a 'flat back'.

In actual fact, the 'flat back' that is so sought after by cyclists requires a nice smooth curve (rather than being literally flat), such that the stress of the position is shared across all the vertebrae, rather than shifting up or down to the junctions at the neck or lower back.

Often, where the thoracic spine is stiff and rigid, the cervical spine begins to suffer. A stiff upper thoracic spine can cause neck pain because where some joints become stiff those above often become hypermobile or loose.

If postural changes at the upper thoracic spine and neck junction are not addressed, over time bony changes can begin to occur as the body attempts to provide more stability. These 'arthritic' changes are irreversible and for cyclists can lead to poor mobility at the neck in the cycling position and lasting pain issues that become difficult to work around.

Where thicker 6-inch diameter foam rollers are useful for massaging muscle and tissue, a 4-inch diameter foam roller is best for mobilizing the spine because when you lie across it horizontally, the apex of the curve is better suited for separating the vertebrae.

Foam rollers have in recent years become widely available in gyms and rehab settings for 'self-massage'. In practice, different widths of rollers and other myofascial release tools are good for different muscles or areas. Most gyms provide thick 6-inch diameter rollers, most useful for rolling and releasing large muscle areas like the thighs, hips and large latissimus dorsi muscles of the back. Tennis balls and other balls of various sizes are useful for getting to more specific tight spots, like deep into the buttock or into the calves. Their sharper apex can also help identify 'trigger points' or 'knots' in the muscle that need focused work. A firm 4-inch diameter foam roller is ideal for working across the upper back to encourage and maintain mobility of the vertebrae. A 6-inch diameter roller is not because it's broad enough to cross several joints of the spine and will therefore be relatively ineffective at mobilizing each one in turn.

Longitudinal foam roller mobilization (and pec stretch)

This first 'longitudinal foam roller mobilization' can be done lying lengthways along a 4-inch or 6-inch diameter roller. The 6-inch diameter rollers are more widely available in gyms. However, the 4-inch foam roller is needed for the 'horizontal foam roller mobilization' that follows.

Preparation

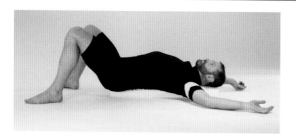

Lie lengthways along the roller with your knees bent and your feet hip-width apart. Make sure that your hips are on one end and your head is on the other. Focus on breathing deeply into your abdomen so that it rises up on the in breath. If you struggle with this, place one hand on your abdomen and the other on your chest. As you breathe in deeply, your abdomen should fill with air first. Only then with the final part of a full deep breath should your chest rise up.

The importance of breathing correctly

This deep diaphragmatic breathing is really important in establishing normal breathing patterns and in maximizing gains from all the stretches that will follow in this section. For many people who are stressed out on a daily basis, an 'inverted' breathing pattern can develop where the chest rises first together with the shoulders coming up around the ears. This is not normal relaxed breathing, and can contribute to neck tension and headaches by way of overworking the accessory respiratory muscles around the neck.

If you find the breathing pattern described difficult, don't worry. If you take time out daily to practise, it will gradually become easier and the benefits to your body as a whole will be enormous.

Introductory pec/shoulder stretch

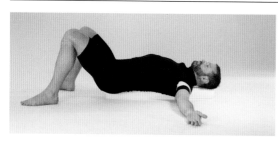

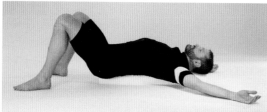

Once you are breathing correctly, relax your arms out to the sides at roughly 90 degrees to your body as shown above left. This preparatory position, together with the deep breathing, helps to open up the ribs and stretch the larger chest muscles too. If you arc your arms upwards (shown below left) you may find a more intense stretch position still.

Bend your elbow to 90 degrees (shown opposite top) and you will be able to stretch the smaller of the pec muscles at the front of the shoulder and the internal rotators of the shoulder too. If the muscles of the rotator cuff of the shoulder are tight, you will find that your forearm sticks up in the air slightly and will not fall naturally to the floor. Just allow the weight of your arm to develop the stretch, working into any areas of tightness, and over time you will find that your arm naturally drops a little lower.

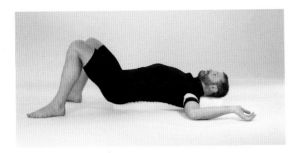

At the front of the shoulder is a group of nerves collectively called the 'brachial plexus'. They originate from the neck and run underneath the collarbone and then down your arm. If you have a rounded upper back and tight chest and neck, you may feel some tingling in your fingers and along your arms in this position as these nerves are being stretched. If this becomes too painful, move your arms a little lower. A moderate stretch to the nerve may lead to this tingling sensation but should not cause any real problems.

Movement – Longitudinal rotational mobilization

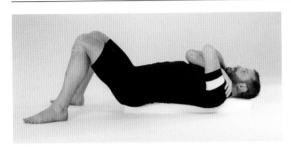

To mobilize your spine in rotation, place your arms across your chest and, working in time with your breathing, turn your shoulders and head one way, and drop your knees the other as you breathe out.

Relax as long as you can at the end of the out breath before returning to the centre position as you breathe in, and then twisting in the opposite direction on the next out breath. Ensure that the roller supports your head as you twist your body to avoid any neck discomfort or tension.

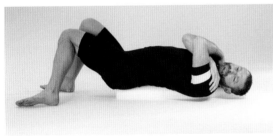

Initially this rotation on the roller can seem a little unsteady, and you may find that you fall off or wobble a lot, and that you struggle to coordinate the movement and the breathing together. With practice, as you learn to counterbalance the upper and lower body movements you will gradually be able to integrate the breathing pattern more effectively into the movement. Resting your elbows on the floor when you begin to learn the twist can help if you are finding it really difficult. Dropping into the twist on the out breath really helps to maximize the impact of the exercise, so persist with the practice, first learning the breathing and twisting separately before trying to bring them together at the same time.

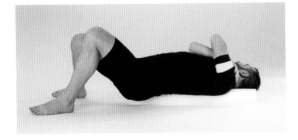

When and how much?

Pre-exercise: Perform 12–16 alternating rotations slowly. This should take you approximately 2 minutes.

Post-exercise: Spend 2–5 minutes in the various pec stretching positions, focused on finding tight spots and letting go of them progressively with every out breath. Then spend 2–5 minutes on the longitudinal rotations, breathing for 12–20 alternating rotations, or until you feel relaxed and more mobile through your spine and upper back.

This exercise can be quite relaxing and can be performed daily if you feel better for doing it and know you are stiff in your upper back. Including it regularly at weekends after your longest rides can prevent problems developing from the postural strain of being on a bike for hours at a time.

Horizontal foam roller mobilization

Preparation

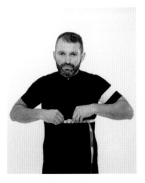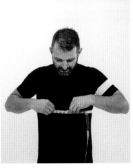

This next foam roller exercise is more vigorous than the last and requires a minimum level of rib and spine mobility to be safe and effective. To test that you are ready for this exercise, run a tape measure around your chest (as you would a heart rate monitor) and exhale completely to draw the tape tight. Then take a deep breath in, and measure whether you are able to expand your chest by 2 inches (about 4–5cm). If you find you are not easily able to expand your ribs in this way, keep working on the previous longitudinal exercises and intermittently retest your rib expansion to see if it has improved (Magee, 2008).

Movement

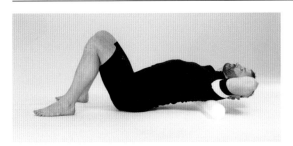

Lie on the roller with it across the top of your upper back, but not on your neck. Support your head with your hands interlocked behind your neck creating a kind of neck 'brace'.

Keep your knees bent with your feet flat on the floor to prevent too much strain on your lower back. Take two or three deep diaphragmatic breaths in this position, focusing on 'letting go' onto the foam roller as you breathe out. The more relaxed you can be, the more effective the mobilization.

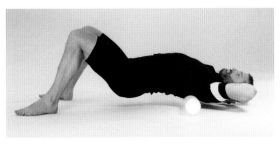

Push with your legs, lifting your hips off the ground as you move over the roller, until the roller is positioned slightly lower down your back.

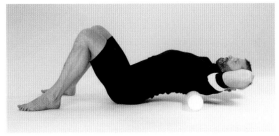

Drop your hips, relax as much as you can and take several deep breaths. Move slowly, inch by inch and avoid making big movements along the roller. Your goal is to ensure you have mobilized all the joints along the thoracic spine.

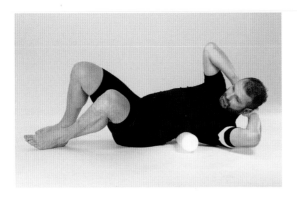

Repeat this movement all the way down your upper back until the roller is opposite your lowest ribs (but not on your lower back). When you have worked down the spine in this way, roll off sideways (rather than sitting straight up). If you are stiff in this area, this mobilization can be quite uncomfortable to start with. Any time it becomes too uncomfortable, roll off sideways. By doing what little you can as often as possible, it will begin to get easier.

Once you are comfortable working top to bottom with this exercise, you can work in the opposite direction, pulling your body over the roller as you lift your hips, working from opposite your lower ribs up towards your neck. Moving in this direction has the benefit of gently 'tractioning' your spine every time you move and pull, and can be a good addition once you have mastered the basics.

Performing the longitudinal and horizontal foam roller mobilizations together will give you the biggest benefit, since the breathing and rotation of the first exercise is an effective preparation for the extension of the second.

When and how much?

Pre-exercise: Work from top to bottom, taking two to three deep breaths on each of six to eight spots as you work from the upper back towards your waist. This should take you approximately 2–3 minutes.

Post-exercise: Work top to bottom and then bottom to top, first lifting your hips and pushing yourself over the roller, before lifting and pulling to gently traction the spine as described above, moving in the opposite direction. If you find certain spots that feel particularly resistant or uncomfortable, try to spend longer on them to target the mobilization to where you need it the most. Spend 4–6 minutes lying across the roller in this way.

This mobilization can be performed anytime but is most useful after a long ride where you have spent many hours bent over the bike, as well as in combination with the previous longitudinal foam roller mobilization. The harder you find this exercise, the more you need it, and a 'little and often' approach will help you make progress.

Mobilizations for the lumbar spine (lower back)

The lower back is often a problem area for cyclists because of the impact that a seated forwards bend has on the joints and structures of the lumbar spine. Cyclists often develop a 'flat back' posture from this prolonged flexion coupled with the pull of tight hamstrings attaching at the sitting bones of the pelvis.

You will get the most benefit from these lower back stretches by mobilizing the thoracic spine in rotation and extension first, but if you have good thoracic movement or are short on time and your lower back is a priority, you can start here.

Mobilizing the joints and structures of the lower back before stretching the muscles that surround it will help to maximize the benefits of the stretches. However, because of the forward bend on the bike and the shortening action of the hamstrings, it is wise to look closely at the hamstring stretches in this section too if you have any history of lower back problems.

The chances are that if you have lower back pain you will also have short and tight hamstrings. Combining the back mobilizations here with the hamstring stretches later on will give you the best chance of having a significant impact, as well as achieving an optimal position for power and performance.

In some cases, your 'bike fit' (the way you have set up your bike) can contribute to lower back problems. Ensuring that your weight is poised and balanced between your saddle, the handlebars and the pedals should create a gentle 'tractioning' effect on the lumbar spine. It is a common misconception that a 'higher' front end (with little or no 'drop' or reach to the handlebars) protects a vulnerable back, when in fact it often provokes it by increasing lumbar compression.

If the stretches and mobilizations in this section fail to have an impact on your lower back, you should consider taking a closer look at your bike fit. A detailed discussion of the biomechanics of bike fit is outside the scope of this book but is highly relevant when it comes to minimizing postural stress on the spine, as well as maximizing effective range of motion of the muscles involved in the cycling action.

In my opinion a good bike fit will look at the body and the bike together, and make recommendations as to how to adjust both. I have been involved in a bike-fitting service for several years now and have found that many clients who come for a fit also need exercises to improve the biomechanics of their body to adapt or improve their cycling position. A body assessment as part of a bike fit should come in two parts – the elements of the body that don't change (such as limb length, proportions and height), and those elements that can change (such as flexibility, mobility and core control). Recommendations as to how to improve both will have the biggest positive impact. Some riders who come for a bike fit expect changes in the bike set-up alone to completely resolve long-standing issues that have developed in their body. While a good bike fit certainly helps, if you have muscle imbalances that have developed over many years you will need to address these with appropriate exercise in order to achieve an optimal cycling position.

The McKenzie press-up

The McKenzie press-up is a simple exercise designed to mobilize the lower back gently into extension while at the same time encouraging the lumbar discs to centralize. With the progressive lumbar flattening that is common in cyclists, there can also be a loss of movement in extension (backwards bending), together with a gradual migration of the lumbar discs in a posterior (backwards) direction.

The goal throughout this exercise is to remain 'passive' through the lower back, avoiding any contraction of the muscles of the lower back and glutes. It should not be confused with similar Pilates- and yoga-style exercises where the mid-back muscles are actively engaged to lift the body off the ground, with some assistance from the arms and upper body.

Preparation

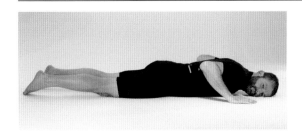

Lie flat on your front with your hands level with your shoulders (but a little wider) and your feet hip-width apart, relaxed and turned in. Place your hands wide enough that you are able to get enough push with your arms and chest to allow your body to be relaxed throughout the process.

Movement

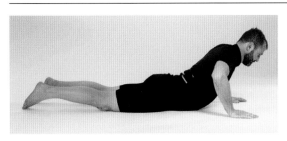

Take a full, deep breath in, and as you breathe out push away from the the floor, making sure you keep your hips, back and buttocks relaxed and 'heavy'. Move slowly, and stop as soon as you feel any tension in your hips/buttocks, or as soon as you feel your hips lifting up off the floor.

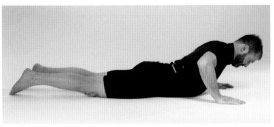

As you lower your body back to the start position, breathe in deeply. You should try to move in time with your breathing, breathing out as you push yourself away from the floor and breathing in as you lower your body back to the floor. Work into the movement progressively so that you are not forcing it, but gradually teasing the mobilization out of your spine.

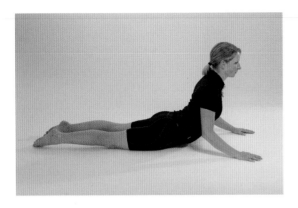

If you are fairly flexible, you may find that you can almost straighten your arms without any tension creeping into your hips, and without too much difficulty.

If you can easily straighten your arms but experience pain in the lower back with this movement, you should leave the exercise out. It may be that you have a tendency towards hypermobility and too much stretching and mobility work will provoke problems. For others, even though you have quite good range of movement, using this exercise intermittently may be therapeutic and feel beneficial. Nichola (left) shows how this exercise will look with good range of movement in the lower back.

When and how much?

Pre-exercise: Perform 8–10 repetitions, or enough to feel more mobile in your lower back. This should take 1–2 minutes. Move slowly in time with your breathing, progressively working your way into the movement and ensuring that your hips remain relaxed. For cyclists whose arms are weaker than their back is stiff, it is perfectly acceptable to break the repetitions into sets of five to give your arms a brief rest.

If you have known lower back problems, you may find that including this exercise first thing in the morning when you are stiffest helps. Move slowly and feel your way into the exercise.

Post-exercise: Perform 8–10 repetitions, or until you feel more mobile in your lower back. After long days in the saddle several sets with a brief rest may be optimal.

Stretching muscles – different approaches pre- and post-exercise

In the next section of exercises we start to stretch muscles or tissue rather than mobilizing joints. There are different methods for stretching muscles 'pre-exercise' as opposed to 'post-exercise', and the confusion around which is appropriate is often given as a reason not to stretch at all. Understanding the key differences that should characterize pre- and post-exercise stretching can help remove this barrier and enable you to effectively use both as appropriate.

Pre-exercise stretches need to be dynamic and held for only moments at a time. In practice, you are often using the muscle opposing the one being stretched to move into the stretch position, and the end range of the stretch will be held only for one or two seconds, before moving away from the stretch.

Sometimes 'active' techniques may also include 'contract-relax' phases where the muscle to be stretched is contracted momentarily before the stretch is repeated. These dynamic interruptions to the stretch itself take advantage of the neurological mechanisms within the joint to try to facilitate and enhance the stretch.

Collectively known as 'proprio-neuromuscular facilitation' techniques (PNF), they take advantage of stretch receptors within the joint that detect high levels of tension and reciprocally inhibit the muscle being stretched to avoid it becoming injured. In simple terms, the muscle that contracts isometrically (without movement) when stretched will then stretch a little further when the tension is released.

Because the tension needs to be high to stimulate this response, these stretch techniques can feel quite intense for short periods, and consequently will be stimulating rather than relaxing. The pre-exercise Swiss ball quad and hip flexor stretch in this section is a good example of how this works in practice.

Characteristics of pre-exercise stretches/mobilizations

- Should be 'dynamic' and 'short hold', such that you either move into and out of position or use 'contract-relax' techniques to enhance the stretch and stimulate the sympathetic ('fight or flight') side of the nervous system.

- They should leave you feeling more awake and alert, ready for exercise.
- They can be used to reduce the 'tonicity' of 'overactive' muscles so that during your cycling movements or core and strength work you are more likely to engage their often weaker counterparts.

A muscle's 'tonicity' is its resistance to stretch during a rested state, or its resting level of contraction. A hypertonic muscle will be more likely to contract in any given movement. A good example among cyclists is where the quads at the front of the thigh can become 'hypertonic', and somewhat inhibit the activation of the glute at the back of the hips.

Post-exercise stretches should be more relaxing in nature and can be held for longer periods. Since the body is not preparing itself for activity, the more passive you can be the more effective the stretch will become, and you will be able to comfortably hold positions for longer, allowing time for the muscle to 'let go' and release.

The intensity of post-exercise stretching can also be more moderate, such that you seek a position that is slightly uncomfortable and then focus on relaxing by way of continuous deep breathing. The doorframe hamstring stretch in this chapter is a good example of a passive, longer hold, post-exercise stretch.

Characteristics of post-exercise stretches/mobilizations

- They should be more 'passive' and 'longer hold' so that you focus on your breathing to 'let go' of the muscle area and stimulate the parasympathetic ('rest and repair') side of the nervous system.
- They should leave you feeling more relaxed and enhance your ability to sleep or rest.
- They are best used to lengthen chronically short muscles or mobilize particularly stiff areas, as well as preventing muscles that have been working hard from shortening between training sessions.

Persistently tight areas will probably need pre- and post-exercise stretching to maximize your progress. If you find that you are very tight in lots of areas when working through these stretches, designing yourself a stretch-only plan may be the best way for you to start.

Stretches for the lower back

Swiss ball side stretch

This stretch targets the muscles of the lower back as well as the trunk/abdomen. Often, stretches for the lower back involve a forwards bend, but because cyclists are 'flexion dominant' I believe it's more effective to target one 'side' at a time with a sideways bend that helps open up and isolate each side of the body individually. This also ensures that both sides of your back are stretched effectively and that you are able to identify and work on any asymmetries you may notice in your body, comparing one side to the other.

For some riders who have turned to cycling after playing a one-sided sport such as tennis or golf, shortness on one side of the lower back relative to the other can cause pain and problems sitting in the saddle and bending forwards to reach the bars.

If this describes you, you will feel discomfort predominantly on one side of the lower back when riding, usually on the tighter side. This problem can be corrected by ensuring that tightness on one side is addressed and balanced first, before working on stretching both sides in a more equal way.

If you know that you are tighter on one side of your lower back, or you can feel a difference in your flexibility when you perform this side stretch, work on the restricted side more until you feel more equal.

Preparation

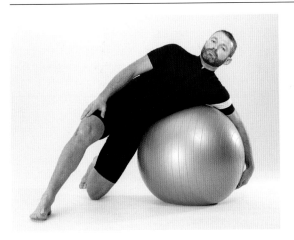

Tuck the ball tight into your side as you kneel next to it in a split stance, one foot forward and the other back behind you. Generally it's easier to balance with the outside leg positioned forwards. Make sure that there is no space between you and the ball, and bring your feet in closely with the toes of your rear foot tucked under ready to push up and over.

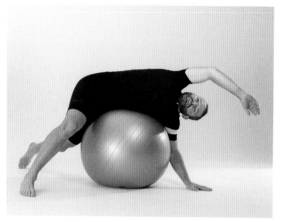

Keeping no space between you and the ball, push up and over the ball using your legs, and allow your body to drape sideways. Try to move far enough that your waist is on the apex of the ball and your head and neck are gently falling down the other side. It's important to relax your head and neck in the position, as the weight of your head and the pull along the oblique muscles down to your waist will facilitate the stretch.

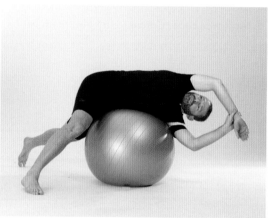

Keep your torso purely sideways over the ball with your hips and shoulders stacked one on top of the other. Try to avoid twisting or rolling forwards or backwards. If you struggle with your balance as you push onto the ball, you can keep your knee on the ground and just lie sideways to start with until you begin to adapt to the movement. If you are comfortable stretching well over the ball, grasp your top arm at the wrist with your bottom arm and pull along the line of your body to enhance the stretch (see left).

When and how much?

Pre-exercise: Push up and over the ball holding a strong stretch at the top for 1–2 seconds 8–10 times on both sides. This should take 2–3 minutes once you have got used to moving around the ball. If you know you are tighter on one side then repeat the stretch more on that side. The typical way to do this is to start with the tighter side and then come back to it a second time after you have switched. Where you know there is an asymmetry in the tightness of your lower back you should prioritize this stretch before riding as it may help to push back the onset of backache during the ride.

Post-exercise: Push up and over the ball and relax, seeking out the areas around your back and torso that need the stretch by going further over the ball, or by allowing your torso to rotate slightly, forwards or back. Hold each position for 20–30 seconds or until the line of tension starts to ease, before changing to a slightly different position. You can spend 3–5 minutes working into the sides of your body if it feels good.

Mobilizations and stretches for the hips and legs

The hips and legs are the muscular engine room for any cyclist and the area where you feel the most tightness caused by the exertion of pushing the pedals for long periods. It's important to keep the hip and leg muscles supple so that you can effectively apply force from the saddle down through each pedal stroke, and also because tightness in the hips can cause neurological issues that may limit power and cause pain.

The prime movers in cycling are the gluteals (buttocks), 'upper' hamstrings and quadriceps muscles on the downstroke, and the hip flexors and 'lower' hamstrings at the knee on the upstroke. Where the glutes and upper hamstrings work in a lengthened position on the downstroke they have a tendency to become weak, while the lower hamstrings, hip flexors and (lateral) quads, working in a shortened position, tend to become tight. Muscle imbalances don't always develop in this way but this is a tendency common in cyclists because of the postural position on the bike relative to our anatomical norm of upright walking or running.

During highly repetitive movements such as cycling, where one muscle becomes short, another opposing or related muscle will often become weak, and if this muscle imbalance progresses, your force potential across that joint will begin to diminish.

Most of the stretches in this section target muscles that are working in their shortened range during the pedalling action (such as the hamstrings at the knee), and others target areas that tend to shorten as a compensation for weaker areas (such as the deep piriformis muscle, which can tighten as the larger glutes weaken).

Later, in Chapter 4, I will show you how to strengthen the weaker parts in these partnerships so that you can bring your body towards better balance and improved performance. Using the pre-stretches in this section before riding can be a first step in correcting these imbalances and immediately improving your cycling performance.

Post-exercise stretching through the tightest of these areas can assist in recovery as well as preventing chronic shortness from developing. The harder you find each of these stretches, the more likely you are to need post-exercise stretching as part of your exercise programme to address chronic tightness.

Piriformis stretch

The piriformis is a small but troublesome muscle that often needs some attention. If you have heard of the piriformis it may be because you have suffered from 'piriformis syndrome', where tightness in the muscle affects the sciatic nerve causing pain, weakness and numbness in your buttock or down your leg. You may also know where it is because a well-meaning massage therapist or physio has dug their elbow deep into your buttock to release it for you. Though this is sometimes necessary and helpful, learning how to release the piriformis yourself is often preferable to the ignominy of having someone else do it.

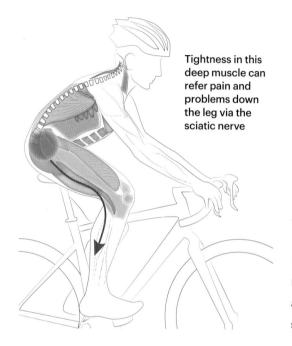

Tightness in this deep muscle can refer pain and problems down the leg via the sciatic nerve

This small, deep gluteal muscle assists in externally or laterally rotating the hip, but can become short and tight when the larger gluteal muscles that should be doing most of the work become weak or inactive. Because of the repetitive, low-load, one-dimensional nature of cycling, the larger glute muscles of cyclists are often weak and underdeveloped, while this smaller muscle can be tight and stiff.

Furthermore, the shortening of the hip flexors at the front of the pelvis that results from prolonged sitting in the saddle can tend to reciprocally inhibit the major glutes and upper hamstrings at the back. Where the lower hamstrings can become short and tight at the knee, the upper hamstrings at the hips also become weak, together with the glutes. When they are strong and functioning well, the glutes are the strongest muscle, contributing significantly to your power by driving hip extension on the downstroke. Take a look at the size of any track sprinter's backside and you will see how effective these big muscles can become at higher intensities.

'Reciprocal inhibition' is a term given to the body's neurological protective mechanism that prevents two opposing muscles from working against each other. A contraction in one muscle inhibits a contraction in its opposing number.

If your piriformis is tight, it may be a sign that your larger glutes are somewhat weak, while this smaller deeper muscle progressively overworks. Most often you will become aware of this only at the point you are having quite debilitating problems, such as neurological pain deep in the buttock or running down your leg. Stretching and mobilizing your piriformis with the exercise described here, together with including some of the glute-strengthening exercises described in Chapter 4 later, will give you the best chance of correcting this imbalance, or preventing it from developing in the first place.

Because the piriformis is very close to the sciatic nerve, often numbness, weakness or radiating nerve pain down one or both legs can develop when it becomes chronically tight. In some people the sciatic nerve actually runs through the muscle, while in most people it runs beneath it.

'Sciatica' is a broad term describing any symptoms caused by compression or irritation of the lumbar and sacral nerves as they exit the spine and run down the legs. 'Piriformis syndrome' is one cause, but lumbar disc 'bulges' and other changes in the functional anatomy of the spine can be implicated too.

If you have symptoms that cause shooting pain, numbness, or pins and needles down your leg, these should be taken seriously and you should find a physiotherapist or osteopath who can assess the cause of the problem. These kinds of problems can stop you riding your bike, limit your power massively (by neural inhibition), and at the very least significantly limit your enjoyment, so prevention is far better than cure.

'Neural inhibition' is a term to describe a mechanism within the body that prevents further injury if nerves are being compressed or joints are at risk. For example, where a nerve that is exiting the spine to serve a muscle in the leg is being compressed, that muscle will appear weak because it is unable to receive the stimulus necessary to contract fully. In this instance, it is not the muscle that is weak, but that the nerve serving the muscle is being affected.

Preparation

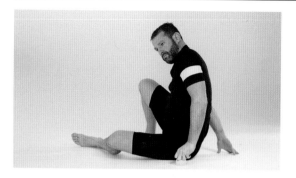

As the piriformis is a deep muscle, you need to relax your buttocks as much as possible to work through the outer gluteals to get to it. Using this simple but effective tennis ball mobilization can help you use your body weight on the ball to locate and work out the tight areas.

Sit on the floor as shown, next to a tennis ball, with your front (left) hip/leg open at a right angle. Use your other leg with your foot flat on the floor, as well as your arms to lift yourself up and sit steadily and carefully back down with the tennis ball centred on your left buttock.

Movement

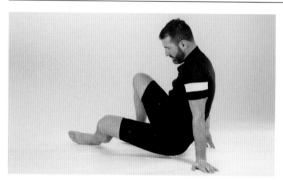

Gradually dropping your weight onto the ball, wriggle around until you feel you are sitting on a tight spot in the area. Generally this will be right in the centre of your buttock. Gently drop your weight onto the ball until it becomes uncomfortable for a couple of seconds. It's important not to tense up but try to relax the leg and hip that you are sitting on. After 1–2 seconds, relieve the tension by lifting your body off the ball slightly. Repeat five or six times until the tension eases, and then move onto a slightly different spot until you have worked through the whole area.

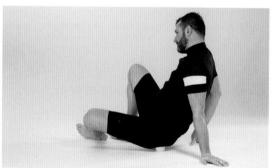

Work into both sides in this way, spending the most time where it feels the tightest. This is an excellent stretch for these little muscles pre-ride and can help you recruit the stronger glute muscles when you get on your bike. Alternatively you can use it to loosen off your hips post-ride. Always strive for equality on both sides, and spend more time on one side if it seems tighter.

How much and when?

Pre-exercise: Spend 2–3 minutes working into the areas on both sides, or until you feel you have released some of the tension. If you know you are tight in this area or have been suffering from 'piriformis syndrome', take particular care with the exercise so that you don't suddenly put a lot of pressure on the focal point of the tightness. If you rush this and are too brutal with it, you may irritate the sciatic nerve, which could make problems worse, not better.

Post-exercise: Use the tennis ball mobilization exactly as described here, but follow up immediately with the wall glute stretch, opposite. If this is a known problem area for you, I would recommend performing both glute stretches after every longer, harder ride.

Wall glute stretch (post-exercise only)

This 'wall glute stretch' offers a post-exercise, more generalized gluteal stretch to the previous piriformis mobilization. It can help maximize the benefits from the tennis ball mobilization and can also be used to prevent soreness from longer, harder rides to aid recovery.

Preparation

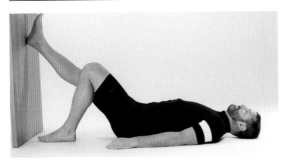

Shuffle up as close to a wall as you can so that both legs are resting on the wall and your hips are able to rest on the ground comfortably and easily. If you set up too close for your flexibility your hips will lift off the floor, if you are too far away, the stretch will be ineffective or impractical as you go into the movement.

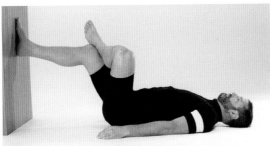

Next, bend your supporting leg and cross the other foot over the knee as shown. Recheck that the distance from the wall is comfortable. If you are too close to the wall your hips will rise up off the floor as you do this.

Movement

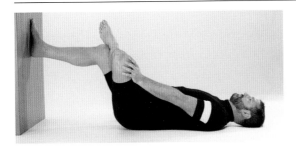

First focus on pushing your tail bone down to the floor. Keep the hips square. Gently push your top knee towards the wall. You will feel a stretch in the buttock. Breathe deeply and relax into the stretch. Hold this position for a minute or longer, before changing sides.

How much and when?

Post-exercise stretching only: The effectiveness of this stretch relies on you taking a little time to locate and work into the tightest area and practise relaxing and breathing into it. If you know you have very tight glutes and feel this stretch deeply, spend 2–5 minutes working from one side to the other, holding each position for a minute at a time before changing sides. If you find that you are tighter on one side than the other, spend a little longer on that side to try to even things up.

Iliotibial band (ITB) foam roller mobilization

The iliotibial band, or ITB as it is often abbreviated, is so called because it runs from the ilium (the crest of the pelvis) to the tibia bone, the larger bone in the lower leg. It is fascia, not a muscle but a fibrous band that wraps around the muscles from the outer hip and along the outer thigh, assisting in extension of the hip (as your leg moves backwards, such as on the downstroke of the pedal) as well as abduction and external rotation (moving your leg out to the side and turning your foot out). Some of the gluteal muscles actually attach to the iliotibial band too.

As a cyclist you may be familiar with the ITB because you have suffered from 'ITB syndrome', which presents as pain in the lateral thigh, more usually towards the knee, or as pain in the knee itself.

The syndrome is an 'overuse injury' in which tightness, stiffness and shortness result in inflammation where the band crosses the knee to attach on the lower leg. Repetitively bending the knee from 30–40 degrees (such as that typical with cycling) is most provocative, together with greater impact or loading (such as when climbing or sprinting hard on the bike). When you go on an intensive training camp where the volume and intensity of riding are both suddenly increased, knee problems can develop as a result.

The ITB is implicated in another syndrome common in cyclists called 'chondromalacia patella' or 'patella femoral pain syndrome'. In this condition the cartilage or underside of the kneecap becomes inflamed, or there is excessive friction as the patella moves up and down the thigh bone.

The long bone of the thigh (the femur) has a groove in it where the kneecap (patella) should smoothly slide up and down as the knee bends. If the tension along the lateral thigh and ITB is too great for the strength of the muscles on the inner thigh the kneecap can be pulled off to one side, causing friction and pain.

Similar issues can aggravate both conditions, and there is considerable overlap between the two. In short, maintaining a flexible and mobile ITB is essential if you want to avoid knee pain of one sort or another as a result of your cycling exploits.

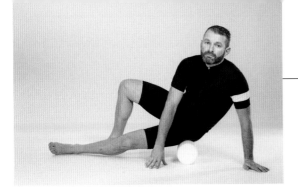

Preparation

Start with your weight resting on the 6-inch diameter foam roller just below your hip on the leg you are going to stretch and mobilize. This bottom leg needs to be straight but relaxed. Use your arms and supporting (bent) leg to take some of the load off the roller so that it is not too uncomfortable.

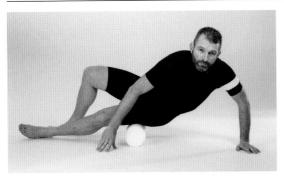

Movement

Moving slowly and managing the intensity of the discomfort with your arms and the supporting leg, start to slowly inch your way over the roller, pushing with your bent leg and using your arms for support. Move slowly from hip to knee in this way, lingering and 'letting go' over any particularly tight spots as you roll over them. Stop just above your knee and then retrace in the opposite direction from knee to hip.

You can repeat this same 'strip' of tissue two or three times, or roll your hips forwards or backwards so that you are slightly on the front or back of the thigh rather than on the side. Focus on the areas where you feel the tightest until they begin to loosen off.

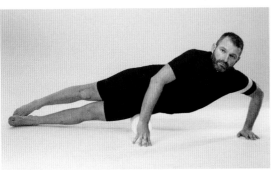

If you struggle to achieve the necessary pressure to be effective, you can work with both legs outstretched and stacked one on top of the other as shown to the left. It is important that the underneath leg remains relaxed in this instance, as it is all too easy to tense up and 'lock out' the muscles.

When and how much?

Pre-exercise: Working along the three 'strips' directly on the side, slightly behind and then slightly in the front, can be a good way to decrease the 'tonicity' in the area pre-ride or prior to other strengthening work. Aim to take approximately 20 seconds from top to bottom and then bottom to top in each of these three areas so that the overall mobilization takes 2 or 3 minutes on each side. If you are tighter on one side than the other spend a little longer on that side. If you have knee problems I highly recommend you use this exercise on a regular basis as it will help you to correct the muscle imbalances at the root of the problem.

Post-exercise: A lot of cyclists are very tight in the ITB, but using this mobilization post-exercise or before bed can have a lasting impact on this persistently tight area. Repeated exposure of 'little and often' works well, as working too deeply too soon can make you sore in the same way that overly zealous deep tissue massage can. This is not a reason to avoid the area, but rather to modify your approach. Try the method suggested for pre-exercise stretching daily, before gradually prolonging the time spent to have a greater impact, provided you do not suffer debilitating soreness as a result.

Swiss ball quad and hip flexor stretch

Most cyclists will be aware of their quadriceps muscles at the front of the thigh. These are the muscles that we feel the most as they fatigue over long rides or hard efforts. The quads are responsible for knee extension (leg straightening) as we push down on the pedals. They need stretching because they work hard as prime movers on the downstroke, but not every quad stretch is created equal, and targeting the most relevant areas of the quads is really important if you are going to prevent imbalances from developing in this important muscle group.

Connected with the quads are the hip flexors, which originate at the spine and pelvis, and cross the hip joint to attach on the long bone at the upper thigh. These muscles flex the hip and are active on the cycling upstroke as we bring our leg up towards the chest.

The 'origin' of a muscle describes where it attaches or 'starts', while the 'insertion' describes where it goes to or 'finishes'. Origins and insertions of muscles are usually on bones but can also be along fascia. The origin is the end of the muscle that usually stays anchored during the contraction while the insertion end moves.

The rectus femoris is one of the four muscles that make up the quads and bridges both the knee and hip, both extending the knee (on the downstroke) and flexing the hip (on the upstroke). Due to this dual action, the rectus femoris muscle can become particularly tight in cyclists as cycling forces the hip end of this muscle to work in a shortened range. For this reason, a quad stretch that also stretches the hip flexors is an essential for cyclists.

In addition to targeting the hip flexors, it's particularly important for cyclists to focus their attention on the lateral part of the quadriceps group, as this tends to become tighter than the medial part. Since the leg remains slightly bent throughout the pedalling action, and the medial or 'inner' portion of the thigh muscles is responsible for the last 15 degrees of knee extension, a discrepancy between 'outer' and 'inner' strength can develop. The vastus medialis, the 'inner' of the four quad muscles, is important in stabilizing the knee joint and weakness here is implicated in knee problems and pain.

For cyclists it's also particularly important to include exercises that stretch the outer quadriceps and strengthen the inner quadriceps. In practice, stretching the outer thighs can be achieved in conjunction with stretching and mobilizing the ITB along the outside of the thigh and hip.

For this reason, the stretch described below is most effective when performed immediately after the ITB foam roller mobilization on the previous pages. It targets the quadriceps group as a whole, but also effectively stretches the rectus femoris at the hip.

Preparation

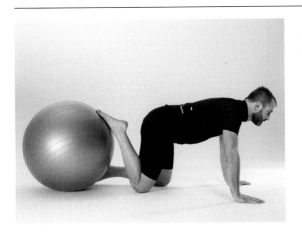

Kneel on all fours in front of the ball, raising one leg up onto it behind you so that the heel of your foot is directly behind your buttock. This exercise is quite difficult to do 'free standing' and it can be helpful to wedge the ball in a corner or up against a sofa so that it doesn't move around too much while you are trying to get into position. In fact, if you are quite tight, this exercise can be performed rather well with your foot up on the seat of a sofa rather than a ball. In this sequence I will show you what it looks like when you are quite tight (as in the case of Paul) and more flexible (as in the case of Nichola), so that you can gauge where you are on the spectrum.

Movement

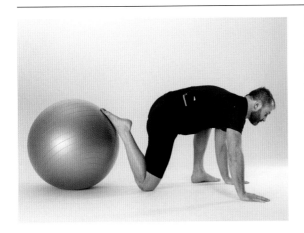

In order to move towards the upright position, slowly move your other leg forwards to place it alongside your hand, or as far forward as you can take it, as shown left. Then, placing both hands on your front knee, slowly push yourself up into the stretch position, drawing your navel in and tucking your tailbone down. The stiffer you are, the harder it will be to bring your body upright, and you may have to have your back knee slightly further away from the ball at the start.

Once you feel the stretch sensation in the quad and hip flexor, hold the position for 1–2 seconds, before kicking your lower leg back into the ball, as if moving from the knee joint. This is an 'isometric' contraction – you are contracting the muscle against an object of resistance but there is no actual movement. By contracting the quads in this way it will momentarily release the stretch sensation.

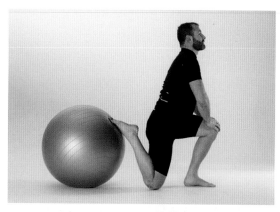

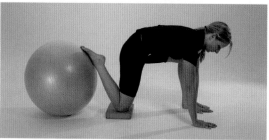

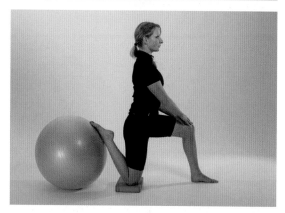

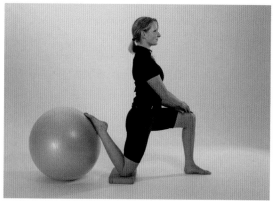

Hold this isometric contraction for 1–2 seconds before releasing the 'kick' and immediately easing further into the stretch, either by gently pushing your body a little more upright as in our stiff example of Paul or by easing slightly forwards as in our more flexible example of Nichola below. Repeat this contract-relax process four to five times or until you are not making any further gains in the movement, before relaxing and changing sides. If you know that you are tighter on one side than the other, come back to the tighter side a second time.

If you are more flexible, you will be able to tuck the knee tighter into the ball at the start and come into a fully upright position much more easily, with the supporting leg brought further forward as seen here. You will also be able to shift forward more easily into the stretch as you work through the contract-relax sequence. Nichola demonstrates the difference with a more flexible quad and hip flexor.

How much and how often?

Pre-exercise: If you are particularly tight in the quads, use the 'contract-relax' method described here for 4–6 repetitions on each side before riding, as well as before any other strength work. This should take you 2 minutes, once you are used to getting into position. This may help prevent the onset of cramp in the quads, or back pain where tightness in the hip flexors is implicated.

Post-exercise: The contract-relax technique can be effectively used post-exercise too, but you can hold the relaxation phase for much longer to allow your thighs to relax for 20–30 seconds before introducing another 'contraction', and then taking the stretch further again. Repeat this method two or three times on each side or until you feel your quads are relinquishing no further. Post-exercise, you can also experiment with positioning the heel of your rear leg more to the centre of your hips or outside of your buttocks to seek out the tightest 'lines' within the quad/hip flexors that you are stretching. This stretch can also be used to prevent soreness from longer, harder rides to aid recovery.

The hamstring stretches

Most cyclists know where their hamstrings are and feel they should stretch them, but many don't know how to do it right, or feel nervous about causing an injury by doing it wrong. Of all the muscle groups that a cyclist ought to learn how to stretch properly, for me the hamstrings come top of the list. Running along the back of the thigh from your pelvis (sitting bones) and down behind the knee, they are a muscle group that can become chronically short and tight in response to sitting for longer than is natural. And that can be sitting in a chair, or in the saddle.

As they originate at the pelvis, when the hamstrings become short and tight they can transfer tension to the lower back in particular (as well as further up the spine) and can be a common causative factor in lower back pain. In cycling-specific terms, shortened hamstrings can also affect your ability to get into an optimal position, especially limiting saddle height and 'drop' from seat to the bars, thereby limiting power production and bike handling. The hamstrings are a muscle group that will always need maintenance stretching as a minimum since the majority of your time pedalling is spent seated, which can encourage tightening.

Most cyclists will have shortened and tight hamstrings at the lower end where the muscles cross the back of the knee. This tension will affect the chain of muscles all the way up the back of the body, but in order to improve muscle balance and your overall flexibility, it's helpful to isolate the stretch to this area to have the biggest impact. This means learning to specifically target your stretch to that lower portion of the muscle.

The hamstrings aren't actually separated into upper and lower, but in terms of how they function the upper portion tends to work with the gluteals to extend the hip, while the lower portion tends to work to bend the knee. For cyclists where the lower portion at the knee often needs stretching, the upper portion at the hip often needs strengthening.

Combining the stretches here, which target the lower hamstrings together with the essential core exercises in Chapter 4, which target the glutes and upper hamstrings will give you the best chance of bringing the muscle group into balance.

I have included several options here to ensure that you will find at least one stretch that you can do effectively and easily. Follow the instructions for each and try them all before deciding on which will be most useful for you.

Supine knee extension

This supine knee extension stretch is the simplest of the dynamic 'pre-exercise' hamstring stretches and doesn't require a strap or belt.

Preparation

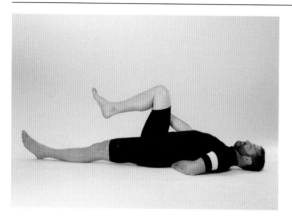

Lie flat on your back, raise one leg and grasp it at the back of your thigh as shown. Your knee should be held directly above your hip with your lower leg relaxed so that your heel drops down. Slide your other hand under your lower back so that you can feel whether your back is rounding and pressing down into the floor as you go into the exercise. In this preparatory position, focus on gently arching your lower back to make room for your hand, and at the same time press down the straight leg at the back of the knee.

Your goal is to maintain a slight curve in your lower back (as assessed with your hand) in order that you target the stretch most effectively to the lower hamstrings behind the knee. Don't allow your back to flatten or your hips to lift as you go into the stretch or the effective position will be lost.

Movement

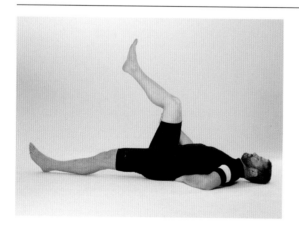

Slowly extend your leg directly upwards, keeping your foot relaxed and focusing on maintaining a curve in the small of your back. As you move into the stretch feel for the point where if you go any higher you will be unable to maintain this curve, at which point hold the stretch position for 1–2 seconds. Then release the lower leg back down relaxing the hamstrings but maintaining the knee-over-hip position.

If you are performing the stretch well you will feel the focal point at the back of the knee. It can take some time to learn to maintain the curve of your back while at the same time extending your leg, but if you persist your control in this exercise will improve, as will its effectiveness. If you have practised but still struggle to feel the stretch in the target area you might want to try the next strap-assisted hamstring option to help you achieve the necessary pressure in order to feel the benefit.

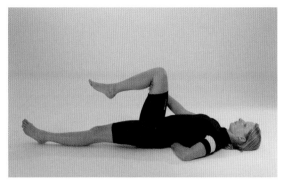

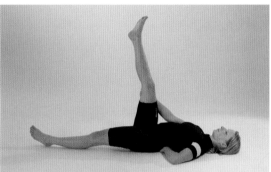

Focus on the 'feel' of the stretch rather than trying to reach your leg high. Paul's leg (previous page) is not fully extended but that is where he can feel the stretch. Here, Nichola shows a greater flexibility in her hamstrings performing the same stretch. She is more able to maintain a neutral curve in her lower back as she extends the leg, and nearly fully extend the knee. This is an example of optimal range in the hamstrings at the knee. Cyclists should aim for extending their range of hamstring flexibility to be confident that their hamstring length does not have a negative impact on bike fit or cycling biomechanics.

When and how often?

Pre-exercise: If you have any lower back problems that are provoked by riding, I highly recommend you include this or any of the other dynamic hamstring stretches before you get on the bike, as well as before any strength or core-focused work. Perform 8–10 repetitions on each side, or more if you feel you need a little longer to start to loosen up in the stretch. You should find that your range increases slightly as the muscles warm up but then will plateau, at which point you will probably not get any further benefit from the stretch.

If you are tighter on one side (which will be evident if one leg does not extend as easily as the other), perform further repetitions on the tighter side until you feel more even. One of the key benefits of this stretch is that you don't need any equipment at all so you can include it anywhere at any time, even if that is before you leave work for your commute home from the office.

Post-exercise: This stretch can be used in this same way post-exercise, but for more repetitions – for example 16–20 on each leg. Post-exercise, one of the strap-assisted options or the longer hold doorframe stretch will probably be more effective if you are particularly tight in this area.

Supine knee extension – strap assisted

This next exercise is very similar to the last, except with the addition of a strap to help intensify the stretch, making it more effective, particularly if your hamstrings are very tight and don't respond to stretching easily. (I adapted this technique from the version I learned from AIS practitioner Hughie J Morris.)

Preparation

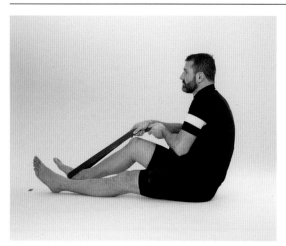

Hook a strap around the instep of your foot. The strap needs to be solid (not elastic) and long enough to work with comfortably. In these pictures Paul is using a martial arts belt.

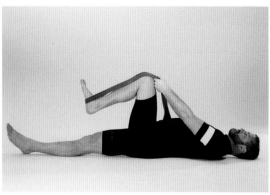

Lie flat on your back and raise one leg directly above your hip, holding the belt at the knee with both hands (shown). Your lower leg should be relaxed. Relax the straight leg down at the back of the knee.

Your goal is to maintain a slight curve in your lower back in order that you target the stretch most effectively to the lower hamstrings behind the knee. Don't allow your back to flatten completely or your hips to lift as you go into the stretch or the effective position will be lost.

Movement

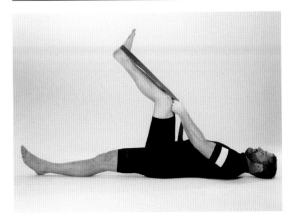

From this start position, slowly extend your leg directly upwards, keeping your foot relaxed and maintaining a curve in the small of your back. As you move into the stretch, feel for the point where if you go any higher you will be unable to maintain this curve, at which point pull firmly on the strap to increase the stretch sensation, and hold for 1–2 seconds. Using your knuckles against your knee as a solid anchor point can help you find and hold the effective position repeatedly. Then, release your lower leg back down to the start position, relaxing the hamstrings but maintaining the knee-over-hip position.

If you are performing the stretch well, you will feel the focal point at the back of the knee. It can take some time to learn to maintain a curve in your lower back while at the same time extending your leg, but if you persist your control in this exercise will improve, as will its effectiveness. It's important that you focus on the 'feel' of the stretch rather than trying to get your leg higher than is optimal for you at any time.

When and how often?

Pre-exercise: If you have any lower back problems that are provoked by riding, I highly recommend you include this or any of the other dynamic hamstring stretches before you get on the bike as well as before any strengthening or core-focused work from Chapters 3 and 4. Perform 8–10 repetitions on each side, or more if you feel you need a little longer to start to loosen up in the stretch. You should find that your range increases slightly as the muscles warm up but then will plateau, at which point you will probably not get any further benefit from the stretch.

If you are tighter on one side (which will be evident if one leg does not extend as easily as the other), perform further repetitions on the tighter side until you feel more even.

Post-exercise: This stretch can be used in this same way post-exercise but for more repetitions – for example, 16–20 on each leg. Following up with the doorframe stretch will be most effective if you are particularly tight in this area.

Activated isolated stretching (AIS) style – strap assisted

This hamstring stretch together with its variations can help you access the different muscles that make up the hamstrings group, and can be particularly helpful if you tend to have neurological symptoms associated with tight hamstrings, such as sciatica or tingly, niggling problems in the hips and legs. The repetitive elevation of the straight leg involved in this stretch can have a nerve-gliding effect, helping to relieve any tethering and tension that can be implicated in these problems.

Preparation

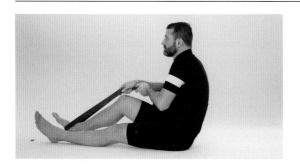

Hook a strap around the instep of your foot. The strap needs to be solid (not elastic) and long enough to work with comfortably. Lie flat on your back with both legs straight, holding on to the leg to be stretched through tension on the strap.

Movement

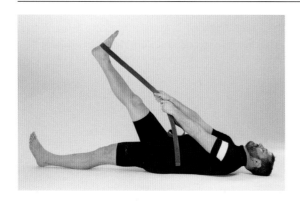

Take a deep breath in and as you breathe out begin to raise your leg, actively using your hip flexors and simultaneously pulling on the strap with your arms. Press the straight leg down at the back of the knee to anchor your hips. At the same time try to release your lower back into its natural curve. Try not to allow your back to flatten completely or your hips to lift as you go into the stretch, or the most effective stretch position will be lost.

Raise your leg to the point where you feel a stretch at the back of the knee, using your quads to keep your leg straight and pulling on the strap with your arms to intensify the stretch. The stretch feeling should be intense and uncomfortable momentarily, but held only for 1–2 seconds (shown left). Then allow your leg to release to the floor, slowly sliding the strap through your fingers.

Repeat this stretch in time with your breathing, breathing out as you raise your leg into the stretch, and breathing in as you lower it. With progressive rhythmical pulls on the strap, you should find that you achieve greater range of movement as the muscle warms up.

Strap wrap variations – medial hamstrings

This variation uses a wrapping technique at the ankle and a lateral pull on the strap to help target the stretch to the medial (or inner thigh) part of the hamstrings.

Preparation

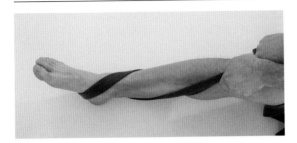

Having hooked the strap around the instep of your foot, take both ends of the strap and wrap them from the outside of your calf to the inside, as shown.

Movement

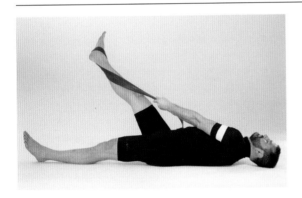

As you go into the stretch movement, raise the leg upwards but also outwards in the direction that your foot is pointing, towards your shoulder, using your lateral glutes as well as your hip flexors. Try to keep your shoulders square and your other hip firmly on the floor by pressing the straight leg downwards behind the knee.

Raise your leg to the point where you feel a stretch at the back of the knee, and/or on the inside of the back of your thigh, using your quads to keep your leg straight and pulling on the strap with your arms to intensify the stretch. The stretch feeling should be quite intense and uncomfortable momentarily, but held only for 1–2 seconds. Then allow your leg to release to the floor, slowly sliding the strap through your fingers.

Repeat this stretch in time with your breathing, breathing out as you raise the leg upwards and outwards into the stretch, and breathing in as you lower it to release the stretch. With progressive rhythmical pulls on the strap, you should find that you achieve greater range of movement as the muscle warms up.

Strap wrap variations – lateral hamstrings

This variation uses a wrapping technique at the ankle and a medial pull (across your body) to help target the stretch to the lateral (outer) part of the hamstrings.

Preparation

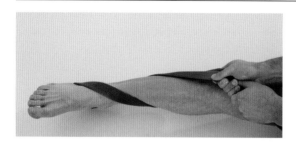

Having hooked the strap around the instep of your foot, take both ends of the strap and wrap them from the inside of your calf to the outside as shown in the picture below.

Movement

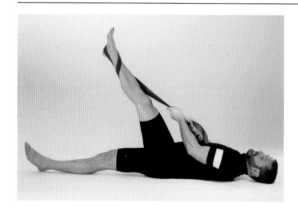

Then as you go into the stretch movement, raise the leg upwards but also inwards in the direction that your foot is pointing, towards your opposite shoulder and across your body, actively using your inner thigh as well as your hip flexors. Try to keep your shoulders square and your other hip firmly on the floor by pressing the leg on the floor down behind the knee.

Raise your leg to the point where you feel a stretch at the back of the knee, and/or on the outside of the back of your thigh, using your quads to keep your leg straight and pulling on the strap with your arms to intensify the stretch. The stretch feeling should be quite intense and uncomfortable momentarily, but held only for 1–2 seconds, before releasing the stretch and letting your leg drop to the floor as you allow the strap to slide through your fingers.

Repeat this stretch in time with your breathing, breathing out as you raise the leg upwards and inwards into the stretch, and breathing in as you lower it to release the stretch. With progressive rhythmical pulls on the strap you should find that you achieve greater range of movement as the muscle warms up.

Working into the tightest areas

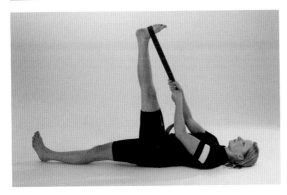

The beauty of this technique is that you can find your way into the tightest spots and compare different angles to target the stretch to where you need it the most.

In this sequence of pictures here you can see Nichola performing the neutral and then medial and lateral stretch variations seen from behind, and with better range of movement than Paul. You can slightly vary the angle of pull to try to find the spot where you feel any restriction and then work into it with progressive pulls on the strap. If you notice that you are not able to raise your leg as high on any particular angle, it is worth performing more repetitions in that plane of movement until you start to loosen up. Balancing the muscles from the inside to the outside, as well as from left to right, can help prevent problems developing.

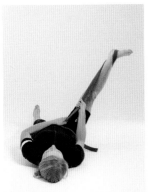 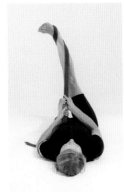

When and how often?

Pre-exercise: If you have any lower back problems that are provoked by riding I highly recommend you include this or any of the other dynamic hamstring stretches before you get on the bike, as well as before any strengthening or core work from Chapters 3 and 4. Perform at least 8–10 repetitions on each side, or more if you feel you need a little longer to start to loosen up in the stretch. You can include at least 8–10 repetitions on all the wrap variations, or just include the angles that you know affect you the most. You should find that your range increases slightly as the muscles warm up but then will plateau, at which point you will probably not get any further benefit from the stretch.

If you are tighter on one side (which will be evident if one leg does not extend as easily as the other), perform further repetitions on the tighter side until you feel more even.

Post-exercise: This exercise can be used in this same way post-exercise but for more repetitions, for example 16–20 on each leg and with each wrap. If you have persistent hamstring tightness and associated problems this dynamic stretch variation can be particularly effective if you spend a bit of time learning the technique and identifying the areas where you are most restricted. Then, you can spend more time post-exercise targeting the angles where you need the stretch the most.

Passive doorframe hamstring stretch – post-exercise only

This hamstring stretch is completely different to those featured so far, as it is entirely passive. That is to say you are trying to relax your leg completely to let the position itself progressively lengthen the muscles. For that reason, it is one of the easiest to do, especially if you are particularly tight. It also works as a good follow up to any of the other more dynamic stretches, and can work particularly well as a relaxation stretch post-exercise, or in the evening.

Preparation

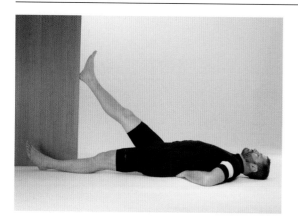

Lie in an open doorway with one leg lying straight through the opening and the other resting on the doorframe or wall.

Position yourself so that the lifted leg is straight and you are able to gently arch your lower back and keep the other leg resting heavily on the floor. You can check you are able to maintain a slight curve under your lower back as shown here by sliding your hand under your lower back.

If you move your hips closer to the wall you will intensify the stretch, move further away and you will ease it. Find the perfect distance for you to be able to let go of your leg but at the same time release your lower back.

Movement

There is no movement with this exercise. You literally just lie there and relax. Focus on taking deep breaths into your abdomen and 'letting go' of the leg resting on the wall or doorframe. The more you attend to letting go of your hamstrings, the more you will release into the stretch.

When and how often?

Post-exercise only: This exercise is an effective post-exercise stretch for developing the length and flexibility of the hamstrings, and also to aid recovery and reduce muscle soreness between longer, harder rides.

The tighter you are, the longer you can hold the stretch position, but a minute at a time before changing sides is a good place to start. You might progress up to 5 minutes on each leg before changing sides, or do five lots of 1 minute on each side, alternating as you go.

It can be tempting to put both legs up the wall to save time, but for most people this position makes it very difficult to keep your hips on the floor and maintain a gentle curve in the lower back, so working on one leg at a time is a lot more effective. If you notice that you are much tighter on one side than the other, then spend longer with the tighter leg elevated to try and bring about balance.

Stretches for neck and upper back

Most riders will report upper back and neck fatigue and aching after a long weekend ride, and for some this can be quite problematic and painful. The postural load of the cycling position on the joints and muscles of the neck is significant, and it's well worth taking care of this area to prevent problems developing, and to make you more comfortable on and off the bike in general. Together with riding a bike, sitting at a desk and working at a computer is very stressful on the neck and upper back, as is using a mobile device, so it's hardly surprising that most people will at the very least suffer a little tension and discomfort here.

Before introducing some simple stretches that help relieve neck tension, it's worth mentioning again that neck problems are often linked to poor posture through the thoracic spine, so I would recommend you look closely at the mobilizations for that area at the beginning of this chapter first. The more mobile your upper back in particular, the less stress will be transferred to the shoulders and neck.

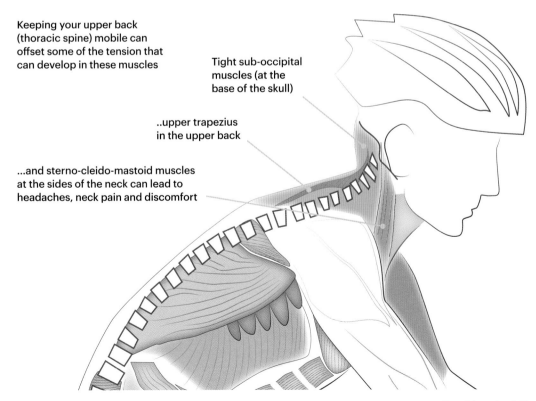

Keeping your upper back (thoracic spine) mobile can offset some of the tension that can develop in these muscles

Tight sub-occipital muscles (at the base of the skull)

..upper trapezius in the upper back

...and sterno-cleido-mastoid muscles at the sides of the neck can lead to headaches, neck pain and discomfort

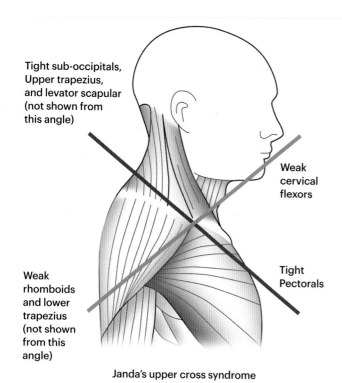

Tight sub-occipitals, Upper trapezius, and levator scapular (not shown from this angle)

Weak cervical flexors

Weak rhomboids and lower trapezius (not shown from this angle)

Tight Pectorals

Janda's upper cross syndrome

Tight neck muscles and poor biomechanics in the neck and upper back can be implicated in recurrent headaches, some neurological problems down the arms, and even dizziness when looking overhead or holding your head in one position for too long. For most cyclists, these problems won't necessarily come to light on the bike at first, but if left unaddressed longer term they can lead to permanent changes in the bony structure of the neck that can have an impact on bike fit and day-to-day movement in general.

The postural 'syndrome' associated with some of these muscle imbalances is known as 'upper-cross syndrome' (Page et al., 2010) where the shoulders are rounded and the head is forwards of the body. Muscles crossing the neck and shoulders front to back are out of balance, with some muscles being over-tight and others being relatively weak. This syndrome is common in cyclists and, as always, stretching and mobilizing the stiff and tight areas before strengthening the weaker areas is a good way to start tackling the problem. Some of the essential core exercises in Chapter 4 will work on the muscles that tend to weaken in this equation.

If you have persistent headaches, neck pain and problems with your shoulders, I recommend you seek out a good physiotherapist or osteopath for assessment and treatment. If you have little movement in your neck but are not in pain, it would be well worth finding a sports or remedial masseur who can do some deep tissue massage in the area. Trigger points ('knots' in the muscle) are very common in the upper back and neck muscles and these won't always respond to the stretches here. However, if you combine them with massage work you will make good progress.

Most people find neck stretches quite uncomfortable, often because the area is so tight; so a little caution in moving into and out of position is worthwhile to ensure you don't aggravate the area in an attempt to improve it.

Upper trapezius neck stretch

The upper trapezius is the top part of the diamond-shaped muscle of your upper back. Although it is one large continuous muscle, in terms of its function the trapezius has three portions: upper, middle and lower. The upper portion elevates the shoulder, and for cyclists supports the upper body when gripping at the handlebars. This upper trapezius makes a coat-hanger-shaped muscle where your neck meets your back, and probably feels tight and tense if you squeeze it with your finger and thumbs.

Most cyclists are tight in the upper trapezius and relatively weak in the mid and lower portions of the muscle. You can very easily see if your upper trapezii are tight by looking at the silhouette of your shoulders in the mirror. If your clavicles (collarbones) are horizontal and level, you are not too tight. If they slope down in the middle your upper trapezius muscles are pulling your shoulders up towards your ears.

Most people will be familiar with the sensation of tension associated with stress here. In situations when you are under pressure, your shoulders may creep progressively upwards around your neck and your breathing may be shallow, moving up towards the chest and neck. Regular, moderate intensity stretching to this area can be the best way to make a start on gently releasing the tension. I have included a stretch seated on the ball here, but you can equally do it sat on a chair, and ideally might repeat it several times a day when at your work desk.

Preparation

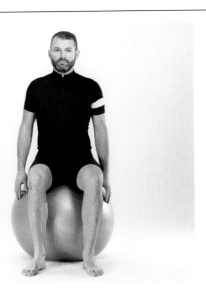

Sit up tall on a chair or ball, lifting your chest and ensuring your lower back is in its natural curve. This will be easier on a ball or chair that is high enough to allow your thigh to slope downwards slightly. Make sure you are not slumping to ensure that your head doesn't fall forwards and is positioned squarely over your shoulders. Your head should be lengthened at the end of your spine so that your ear is directly above your shoulder, if viewed from the side.

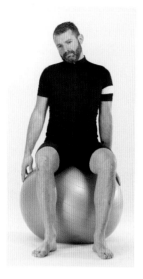
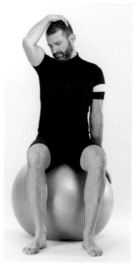

Resting one arm against the side of the chair or ball for reference, keep facing forwards and tilt your head sideways so that your ear drops towards your shoulder. It's important that the opposite shoulder stays down away from your ear as you do this. Lightly gripping the ball or chair on the side that you are trying to keep down can help you get a sense of this.

Next, drop your chin slightly and look down towards your armpit. Keeping your chin tucked close to your chest, lightly grasp the top of your head, and *gently* pull downwards to increase the stretch. Again, focus on keeping the opposite shoulder down away from your ear to ensure you don't lose the effective stretch position. You should feel the stretch in the upper back and neck on the opposite side.

Hold the stretch position for 1–2 seconds only before gently pushing backwards and upwards into your arm. This should be an isometric contraction, meaning that there is no actual movement. Hold the contraction for 1–2 seconds only, before letting go and easing into the stretch a little further, *gently* pulling downwards and across as you tuck your chin in and keep the opposite shoulder depressed.

Repeat this 'contract-relax' process 4–6 times on each side before changing over. Take your time to feel your way into this stretch, 'pushing' with perhaps only 20–30 per cent effort and then seeking out the tight spots as you gently ease into the stretch position.

How much and when?

Pre-exercise: Use the 'contract-relax' method described here for 4–6 repetitions on each side before riding, as well as before any core or strength exercises from Chapters 3 and 4, or at your desk to relieve neck/shoulder tension.

Post-exercise: The contract-relax technique can be effectively used post-exercise too, but you can simply hold the relaxation phase for much longer – for 20–30 seconds. Post-exercise you can leave the 'contract-relax' part out altogether if you prefer and just gently ease into the stretch and hold. Perform several repetitions on each side before changing over. Experimenting with subtle changes in position of the head and neck can help you find the tightest spot that needs the stretch the most. For example, turning your chin slightly more to the right or left may really hit the spot.

This stretch can be quite intense and uncomfortable, and it can be difficult to position the head correctly without your whole upper body moving. Try to be patient in learning the position, and if you are struggling with your head and neck alignment, use a mirror, first to the side and then to the front to help you make sense of what you are doing.

Little and often with this stretch can be most effective as it can help unwind a tense neck and shoulder complex without overstraining or pushing it too far too fast.

Sternocleidomastoid neck stretch

The sternocleidomastoid muscle (SCM) is named after its three main points of bony contact on the body, the sternum (or breast bone), the clavicle (or collarbone) and the mastoid process (a bony prominence on the skull near your ear). Your SCMs are easily visible in the mirror as thick rope like muscles running either side of your throat if you gently tip or turn your head from side to side.

The SCM muscles are involved in almost all movements of the head and neck, and in particular help you to look over your shoulder on the bike and tip and tilt your head to one side or the other. Maintaining good range of movement on both sides of the neck so that you can easily move your head and neck in all directions is important for good visibility on the bike and to stay safe on the road.

Preparation

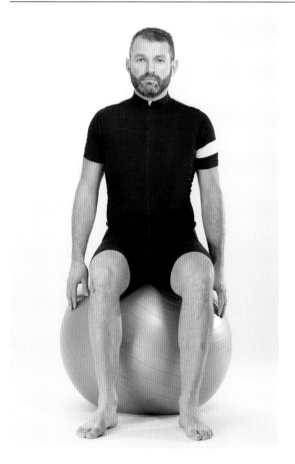

Sit up tall on a chair or ball, lifting your chest and ensuring your lower back is lengthened in its natural curve. This will be easier on a ball or chair that is high enough to allow your thigh to slope downwards slightly. Make sure you are not slumping at all to ensure that your head doesn't fall forwards and is lengthened at the end of your spine and positioned squarely over your shoulders, the back of the head in line with your tailbone.

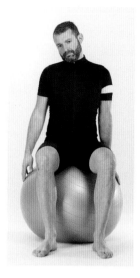 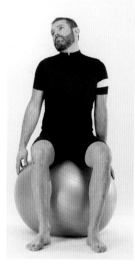

Resting one arm against the side of the chair or ball for reference, face forwards and tilt your head sideways so that your ear drops towards your shoulder. It's important that the opposite shoulder stays down away from your ear as you do this. Lightly gripping the ball or chair on the side that you are trying to keep down can help with this.

Next, tip your head upwards and backwards so that your gaze is directed up and away from your body. This should bring on a stretch sensation in the opposite side of your neck. Hold the stretch position for 1–2 seconds only, before coming carefully out of position to face forwards again.

For this stretch I recommend you hold the stretch position only briefly and check each phase of the movement to ensure you are not accidentally avoiding the effective stretch position. Where the neck muscles are quite tight, it can be difficult to isolate the stretch without your shoulders moving around as a way of avoiding it. By becoming more aware of your seated upright posture you will be more likely to be able to feel the stretch where you are supposed to.

How much and when?

Pre-exercise: Moving into and out of position with care as described, perform 8–10 repetitions on each side before riding, as well as before any strength or core exercises from Chapter 3 and 4, or at your desk to relieve neck and shoulder tension. If you are particularly tight on one side compared to the other, perform more repetitions on the tighter side, or come back to it a second time.

Post-exercise: Post-exercise, this stretch position can be held for much longer. Try holding the position for 20–30 seconds before coming out of the stretch. The stretch sensation should be moderate, not too intense, and repeating 3–4 times on each side will maximize the benefits. Experimenting with subtle changes in position of the head and neck can help you find the tightest spot that needs the stretch the most.

This stretch can be quite intense and uncomfortable, and it can be difficult to position the head without your whole upper body moving. Try to be patient in learning the position, and if you are struggling with your head and neck alignment, use a mirror, first to the side and then to the front to help you make sense of what you are doing.

Little and often with this stretch can be most effective, as it can help unwind a tense neck and shoulder complex without overstraining or pushing it too far too fast.

Essential stretches
ready reference pictures

Longitudinal foam roller pec positions for upper back mobility and chest/shoulder stretch

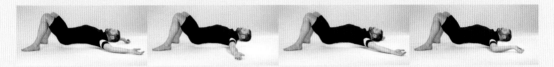

Rotations

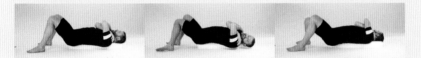

Horizontal foam roller mobilization for upper back mobility in extension

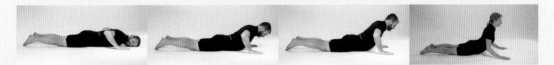

McKenzie press-up for lower back mobility in extension

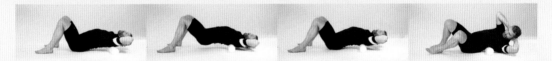

Swiss ball side stretch for the lower back muscles

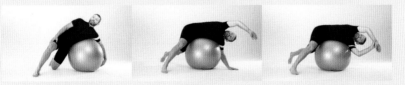

Piriformis mobilization/stretch for the deep buttock and 'sclatic' problems

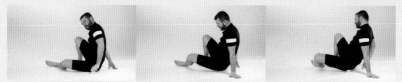

Wall glute stretch for the buttocks as a whole (post-exercise only)

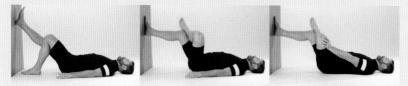

ITB foam roller mobilization for the lateral thigh/hip/knee problems

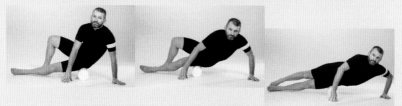

Swiss ball quads/hip flexors for the front of the thigh and hips

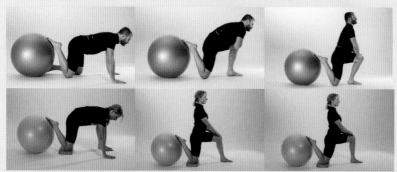

Hamstrings stretches for the back of the thigh and lower back problems

Bent knee free

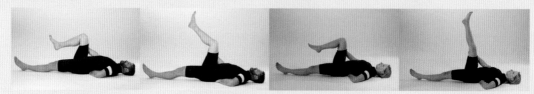

Bent knee strap assisted

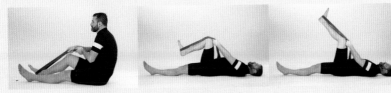

AIS technique strap assisted

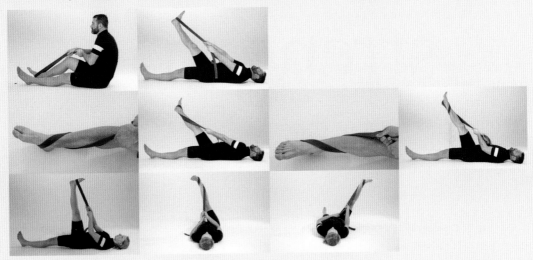

Doorframe passive stretch

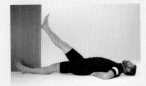

Seated upper trapezius for neck and upper back tension

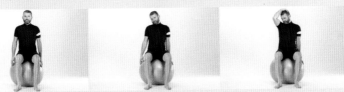

Seated sternocleidomastoid stretch for neck tension

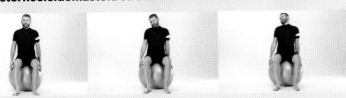

3. Essential strength

Overview of this chapter

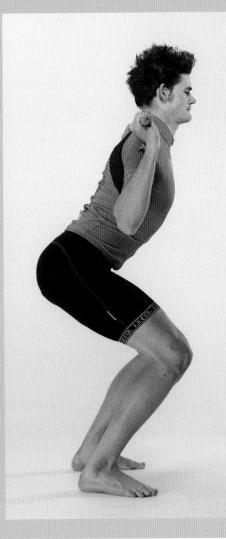

What is strength training and why do cyclists need it?

Hills. Accelerations. Sprinting. These are the strength elements to our endurance sport. These short efforts are what keep you with a group, get you to the top of the hill first, and help you stay out of trouble in traffic. Your cycling strength might be called your ability to generate force through your bike to translate it into road speed. Pure speed may not rely on strength entirely, but when you take into account the time frame during which you are exerting force, that force becomes power.

It's worth remembering that strength is always a prerequisite to power and optimal performance. For cyclists, power has become the trendy measure of performance and can be used as a way to log your progress, and identify and work within your training zones. Your power:weight ratio is the other performance variable that is broadly understood, and for most cyclists the holy grail is to improve power output and reduce body weight.

In this book I refer to 'strength' as your ability to exert force, either on the pedals to move your bike forwards, when using your body weight in an exercise, or when moving weights as part of your conditioning programme. Muscular strength is always a prerequisite to power.

Together with your heart rate, the power you can produce represents a measure of your aerobic capacity: your ability to take in oxygen and use it efficiently. Endurance cycling is predominantly an aerobic sport; that is to say, for the most part your work rate doesn't exceed your ability to take in oxygen and ferry it to the working muscles where it's converted into energy. The bulk of a cyclist's training is focused around becoming more efficient at this 'steady state' type of exercise by way of physiological adaptions in the muscle cells and cardiovascular system.

At low to moderate intensities, where most cyclists spend most of their time, muscular strength doesn't really come into play to any great degree. The work rate from a muscular standpoint is fairly low and so someone with relatively little strength but good cardiovascular fitness can roll along quite nicely on the flat producing good levels of sustainable power. But we all know that cycling isn't like that for very long, and when the road goes up and you start to climb, muscular strength and power become a factor almost immediately, as does your body weight.

Most cyclists will have so many gears on their bikes these days that the strength elements of climbing can be offset quite a lot by changing down to find a comfortable gear and maintaining a higher cadence. However, the benefits of changing down and spinning away have to be weighed up against the speed that will be lost. Having muscular strength at your disposal means that you can push into a hill rather than have it push back at you as you begin to climb. Furthermore, you are more likely to be able to keep that momentum going, or stand up and generate more force out of the saddle if the gradient kicks up further as you approach the summit.

The difference in the feel of climbing as compared to riding along the flat is one of the easiest ways to begin to relate to the strength elements of cycling that we will all encounter. Accelerations and sprints are two other key elements, even if it's only accelerating away from traffic lights, or into or out of a roundabout to try to go with the flow of the traffic. You can of course push harder on the flat too, to make the most of a smooth bit of road, or to chase down another rider ahead of you, and increased muscular effort will be something you will become aware of in these situations too.

The elements of our sport that require more muscular strength include climbing in and out of the saddle, accelerating or sprinting, or pushing harder on the flat. All cyclists need these aspects to one degree or another, and improvements in muscular strength can increase your potential for optimal performance in these areas, as well as making you a more dynamic and responsive rider on the road.

Problems associated with weakness and the benefits of functional strengthening

For many cyclists, this list below will highlight something you recognize you want to work on, and for others it may remind you of things that tend to cause you problems or pain. For example, for many riders an increase in climbing meterage can highlight injury problems and expose weaknesses that went previously unnoticed. Strength will be limited by (in)flexibility and (lack of) core strength in succession, because when the workload becomes challenging muscle imbalances will be exacerbated and your ability to generate force will be limited as a result. Muscles that tend to be short and tight will tighten further, while muscles that tend to be weak or inactive may give up altogether. Understanding that strength needs to be built on good flexibility and a balanced core is essential to make real and tangible changes to your body that will impact on your cycling performance.

Symptoms of weakness

- Poor performance or pain in the strength and power elements of your cycling, including hills, sprints and accelerations in particular.
- Injury off the bike when performing day-to-day functional strength-related tasks such as lifting, carrying or moving objects, children, etc.

Benefits of strengthening

- Potential for optimal performance on the bike, particularly the more dynamic and explosive aspects, with benefits increasing when strengthening is integrated with specific drills and skills as part of a periodized training plan.
- The potential for greater power and change of pace provided by strengthening can particularly benefit competitive cyclists.

A lack of strength can become apparent both on and off the bike in equal measure, but functional strengthening off the bike should be the priority before considering maximizing your strength potential on the bike. Injuries caused by lack of strength in day-to-day activities can prevent the consistency needed in your cycling training that will allow you to move towards integrating sprints, hills and other hard intervals to maximize your performance.

The essential strength exercises in this chapter focus on functional strength first, based around the primal patterns described in Chapter 1. The primary goal of these exercises is to prevent injury that will inhibit your cycling performance.

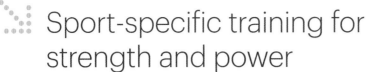

Sport-specific training for strength and power

I discussed some of the arguments for sport-specific training in Chapter 1, and want to reiterate here that it's essential that you train your muscular strength through the cycling movements *on the bike* as part of a year-round periodized programme. Introducing hill repeats, specific muscular drills, sprint efforts and other higher intensity intervals are important for any rider wanting to be the best cyclist they possibly can.

In recognizing the physiological importance of sport-specific training, it's essential to include some on-the-bike strength and power work as part of a periodized training plan, introducing higher intensity intervals as relevant to your cycling goals to maximize the benefits. The secondary goal of the strength exercises here is to develop muscles and movements that have direct carry-over to your cycling. Where there is a direct relationship to these movements, I will make them clear as I introduce each exercise.

Remembering the success formula – knowing where you should start

If you experience pain when climbing, sprinting or pushing hard, I suggest you focus your efforts on the essential stretching and essential core exercises in Chapters 2 and 4, before beginning to introduce some of the essential strength exercises included here. Just skip to Chapter 4 for now.

If you are pain free or have been working on your flexibility and core for some time, you may be ready to include elements across all three aspects in your exercise programme straight away. Chapter 6 on periodization and planning will introduce how you might best include strength exercises as part of your training plan.

Remember the success formula:

FLEXIBILITY
+ CORE STABILITY
+ STRENGTH
= **POWER POTENTIAL**

The primal movement patterns revisited

It may seem illogical but it's quicker, easier and safer to develop strength off the bike first, before integrating that strength into your cycling training. The foundational strength movements that are included here represent a movement vocabulary that every cyclist should learn in order to avoid picking up injuries off the bike, and to allow you to include the higher intensity intervals on the bike that will mean you fulfil your performance potential.

A detailed discussion of on-the-bike strengthening techniques and practices is outside the scope of this book, but they are an essential part of an optimal training programme. I will hint at where these elements fit in throughout Chapter 6. I discussed the relevance of the primal patterns as a basis for strength conditioning cyclists in detail in Chapter 1. In this chapter, I'm going to elaborate on each of these movements further, and then show you how to train them yourself.

For the most part, the exercises here are all the strength exercises you will ever need to get the best out of your riding in the minimum training time. You will be surprised how little you have to do to maintain good posture and have the functional strength to achieve the training effect you are looking for. Furthermore, if you effectively integrate some strength-based cycling drills, intervals and sprints at the right time of year you will see a progressive improvement in your strength-related performance on the bike too, year on year, and aligned with your own personal cycling goals.

Minimal movement requirements to stay healthy

The level of exercise that I am introducing here should represent a minimal standard everyone should aim for in order to maintain musculoskeletal health, fitness and well-being in general. As important as developing the strength in these movements is learning how to move well, so that all sorts of day-to-day tasks can be accomplished with greater ease and efficiency. All movement is neuromuscular, and while the muscular part relates to flexibility and strength working together, the movement part relates to the nervous system, and how it must 'groove' in a consistent pattern that your brain and body can refer to every time you are presented with a movement problem.

Take lifting and carrying, for example. Consider that you want to put your bike up on the roof rack of your car. Several movement patterns will be involved in you achieving this goal. First, you will bend to pick up your bike, before lifting it and pushing it overhead, where you will reach to secure it on the roof rack. When you take your bike off the roof rack, you will go through the same movement patterns in reverse. If you carry your bike in the back of your car, you may have experienced the challenge of bending and reaching to put your bike into the boot, often a more difficult movement, because the weight of the bike is carried further away from your own centre of gravity as you manoeuvre it into position.

As a relatively fit cyclist, it would be very unfair to injure your back putting your bike in your boot as you head off to a big event, but this is not unheard of. Equally, other innocuous household tasks like hoovering or gardening can cause an injury that keeps you off the bike for weeks if you lack strength in these basic movements.

The essential strength exercises in this chapter represent the absolute minimum every cyclist should aim for to avoid injury caused by poor biomechanics, a lack of movement skill, and insufficient strength to perform day-to-day tasks safely. Good technique in the exercises explained here should be achieved before adding more load and weight to develop strength further.

 # Developing your strength further for optimal performance

Some readers may be keen to develop their strength and conditioning further to maximize performance gains. The simplest way to go about this would be to use the exercises in this chapter, but progressively and gradually add load to make the exercises more challenging.

I have deliberately selected exercises here that allow you to learn the movements and begin to load them without any special equipment, aside from a set of adjustable dumbbells that you can keep at home. If you find that using the variations here becomes too easy, it would be worth considering joining a gym so that you have access to heavier weights, as well as more varied ways to train and load the same movements.

The dead lift and the squat in particular need significant loading to maximize the benefits. When you are looking to load more heavily, a barbell can allow you to move more weight than dumbbells can. A squat rack is also a really valuable tool for developing your squat strength to your full potential. Allowing you to load the bar in the rack means that you can carry the weight above your centre of gravity throughout the squatting movement, and don't have the problem of getting the weight into the right position at the beginning and end of the movement. Using the end of a squat rack to perform a dead lift from the top down (rather than from the ground up) can also be useful for cyclists who often struggle to pick a bar up off the floor with a neutral spine to start with. By working from the top down, you can develop strength and flexibility in the movement together, until you have sufficient range to lift safely from the floor.

Another useful tool in a gym environment is a cable machine, which allows you to develop standing strength in pushing, pulling and twisting movements in particular. When working at home your options with these movements are limited, but with a cable pulley you can adjust the direction of pull to almost an infinite number of combinations, offering a more rounded training stimulus and allowing you to combine some of the movements. An example might be a lunge with a single arm push and twist (as shown below).

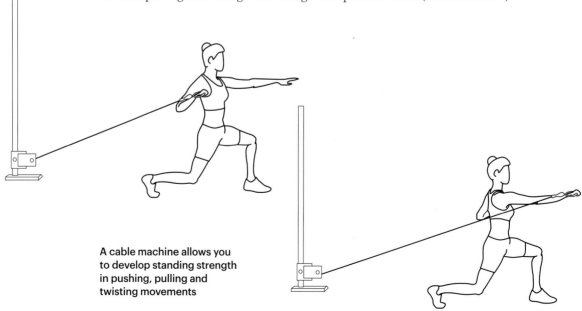

A cable machine allows you to develop standing strength in pushing, pulling and twisting movements

All of these movement options represent just a window into the possibilities that are almost endless if you are interested in exploring strength training further. However, I am conscious that most cyclists prefer to stay out of a gym and can be intimidated by too many choices, which is why I have focused on the essentials here, to give you somewhere to start. The strength essentials in this chapter give most cyclists all they need to stay strong enough to remain injury free and ready to develop the sport-specific strength and power elements on the bike itself. For most cyclists, too many training tools can be a distraction, and going back to basics will keep you focused and ensure that you don't do more than is necessary to achieve your cycling goals in the minimum time.

Whatever level you are working at, 'the form principle' must be applied consciously and consistently. The form principle dictates that you never compromise form for added load. In other words, your position and your technique take priority at all times. You should never be afraid to increase the weight, but you should only do so when you can still maintain good form for the desired number of repetitions. If you follow the technique points outlined in this chapter, and use the photos for guidance, you will achieve good form with the exercises here.

The neutral spine philosophy

Strength is inextricably linked to alignment and muscular balance in the body, and following the form principle is the key to ensuring your alignment is good and you are developing balanced muscles. In a nutshell, if you do a strength exercise well you will get stronger, do it poorly and you may exacerbate imbalances that are contributing to injury and poor performance.

All of the essential strength exercises in this chapter are relatively 'free', and deliberately so. There are no machine weights involved, and they require that you control your body as a coordinated whole, rather than work and develop one muscle in isolation. This more 'functional' approach is key to my approach to conditioning and is explained in more detail in Chapter 1.

Through this chapter you will see that almost exclusively the core maintains a neutral alignment throughout the movement. A neutral spine ready for loading or strengthening

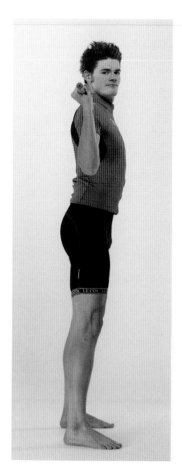

is one where the lower back curves inwards slightly, the upper back is slightly extended with the chest lifted and the head and neck are centred over the body.

Maintaining the natural inwards curve of the lumbar spine when lifting and moving significant load allows the natural biomechanics of the core to do their job. The lumbar discs are able to cushion the load, while the connective tissue of muscles that cross the core assist by decompressing the spine when the abdominal muscles are engaged correctly.

The 'neutral spine philosophy' dictates that whenever you are lifting with significant load (such that you can lift no more than 16–20 reps), you should maintain the natural postural curves of the spine.

For some of you there will be no problem maintaining a neutral spine through the exercises here, while for others it may be more difficult. Squatting and bending movements in particular may take some learning and particular care might need to be taken with the dead lift (bend) movement under load to ensure that you learn correct form. If you struggle to achieve the correct position with the movements here, it's likely that either tightness or poor core control are making it difficult for you to achieve.

Straight vs neutral: Although you may have heard the word 'straight' as a technique cue when exercising, the spine should never actually be straight. The postural curves are dynamic and can change with movement, but an upright spine is more correctly described as 'neutral' because the natural anatomical curves help the body function when loaded from this position.

If in working through the instructions and exercises here you feel you are unable to achieve good form and a 'neutral spine', simply leave the exercises out that you are struggling with, and come back to them at a later date to see how you are doing. If you continue to work on your essential stretches and core exercises you will find your ability to perform these strength exercises improves since the elements of flexibility, core and strength are inextricably connected.

Consciously engaging your core through the strength movements

Maintaining a neutral spine through the movements is very important, but equally important is engaging your core muscles to 'offload' and support your spine in the way described above. For some people core engagement comes naturally and happens automatically, while for others conscious engagement of the abdominal muscles in particular is essential to achieve the desired result.

For most people focusing on 'drawing the navel in' is a useful cue to ensure that the deeper abdominal muscle is engaged and supporting the spine through the movement. If you have already worked through some of the core essentials in Chapter 4 you will most likely have become aware of this core engagement through some of the exercises there. Because the essential core exercises are more 'isolated' you are more likely to get a feel for core engagement, and then be able to maintain that same core control in the more integrated movements here.

If you struggle to get a sense of engaging your core or find it difficult to maintain a neutral spine through the strength exercises here, you might be wise to maintain some of the core essentials in Chapter 4 as part of your programme. As the control and strength of your core improves you will notice the difference that it makes to your ability to perform the strength essentials here.

The impact of short and tight muscles on form and alignment

As well as needing to engage your abdominal muscles throughout the movements, you may find some movements are limited by shortness and tightness too. Two good examples from this chapter are the dead lift and the split squat.

For the dead lift, in order to maintain a neutral spine to strengthen the lower back, gluteals and the upper hamstrings, you have to learn to tip your pelvis down at the front and up at the back as you pivot from the hips into and out of the movement. This ensures that you don't 'round out' your lower back, which can lead to injury, especially under

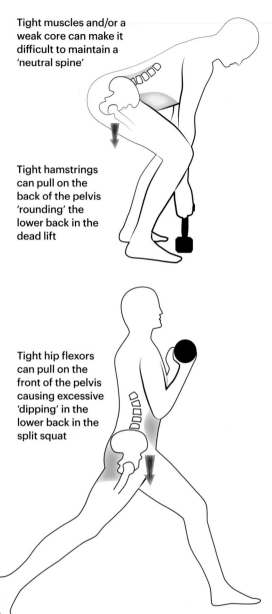

Tight muscles and/or a weak core can make it difficult to maintain a 'neutral spine'

Tight hamstrings can pull on the back of the pelvis 'rounding' the lower back in the dead lift

Tight hip flexors can pull on the front of the pelvis causing excessive 'dipping' in the lower back in the split squat

heavier loads and if the abdominals are not engaging properly. If you have tight hamstrings (as is common in most cyclists) as you get into this position, you will experience a stretch sensation as your tight hamstrings want to pull in the opposite direction, down at the back of the pelvis as you bend forwards. Applying the form principle to this example and only working within a range where you can maintain a neutral spine will help you develop strength in the dead lift and flexibility in your hamstrings at the same time.

In contrast, to achieve and maintain the neutral spine desirable in the split squat you have to learn to consciously tuck your pelvis down at the back to engage the glutes on your back leg to ensure you don't 'dip' into your lower back. If you have short or tight hip flexors at the front of your hip and thigh, as you go into this movement they will tend to pull down on the front of the pelvis, causing this excessive inwards curve in the lower back, and you will have to choose a level of the exercise where you have good control of your pelvis and lower back to move forwards.

Both of these examples show how flexibility is linked to strength, and how working on flexibility and strength together can help you make the most progress. The instructions alongside each of the exercises here are designed to help you achieve the best form possible, even if you have some tightness in some of these areas.

In practical terms, using the essential stretches in Chapter 2 directly before your chosen strength essentials will maximize your chances of optimal form throughout the exercise.

Combining the essential stretching, strength and core exercises in an all-round programme will give you the best chance of improving your all-round condition and cycling performance. Choosing exercises to get the balance right for you will be discussed further in Chapter 6 on programme design and periodization.

Strengthening the upper body

Cyclists often make the mistake of selecting pushing and pulling movements in isolation, believing that the legs and lower body will have developed some strength through cycling. While relatively isolated upper body exercises can be useful for the purposes of balancing or correcting for weakness, overall this rationale is misguided, and doesn't help you develop the functional strength you need day-to-day, to prevent injury and enhance performance. When cycling, the upper and lower body are constantly working together, connected by the core, both seated in the saddle, where the legs are moving and the upper body is stable, and in particular out of the saddle, where both upper and lower body are working connected by an active core.

Working exclusively with isolated upper body exercises (where the lower body is inactive) does little to stimulate the core and does not teach your body to integrate the use of the legs with the arms in real-life situations, and when working harder on the bike, when the upper body becomes more active. For some people (men in particular), this more isolated approach may also lead to unwanted muscle development and weight gain without any added performance benefits.

For these reasons, my first choice of upper body exercises would be standing pushing and pulling exercises where the legs and core are working together with the upper body to generate force. In a gym situation a cable machine is the perfect tool for these exercises, and pushing, pulling and twisting variations can be combined with squatting, lunging, twisting and bending to develop functional upper body strength and flexibility without developing unnecessary bulk.

Since the essential strength exercises in this book are designed to allow you to make a start at home, I have chosen the best upper body strengthening exercises I can using only a ball and dumbbells. As a result, these are relatively isolated exercises compared to the 'primal standard', but they will help to improve your posture and correct for typical weak areas to establish some foundational basics as a minimum standard for upper body work, or as a foundation for further progressions later on.

Repetitions, sets and rest periods

Throughout this chapter you will find that there is some similarity in the number of repetitions, sets and rest periods that I recommend. For strength training enthusiasts and specialists, the science and art of reps, sets and rest periods is quite complex. Depending on what type of strength you are trying to achieve in a particular movement or muscle group, you can manipulate these variables for different and desired results.

A detailed discussion of the science of intensity, repetitions, sets and rest periods is outside the scope of this book. In this chapter on essential strength exercises I have focused on how the exercises should be performed and taken a standard and basic approach to these variables. This is adequate for most cyclists to achieve their goals. For those exploring strength training further, I recommend you find a good personal trainer or strength and conditioning coach who can help you develop a more tailored programme.

With most of the exercises here, there are one or two preparatory exercises to ensure you learn correct form before adding any load. Then, for the most part, I am recommending 8–12 repetitions for each exercise for 2–4 sets, with 1 minute's rest in between sets. In practice, this means that you should be able to do between 8 and 12 repetitions of the exercises with good form, having to concentrate and work hard to maintain your position and technique for the last two or three repetitions. Essentially, you should start to fail between 8 and 12. You should not be able to do more than 12 repetitions, so if you can you need to increase the loading by adding more weight, or choose one of the more challenging versions of the exercise. If you are unable to do eight repetitions with good form, you can either choose an easier version of the exercise, or leave it out altogether until your core strength and flexibility improves.

The level of the exercises and the number of sets suggested here should help bring about strength without adding much muscular weight. For some individuals there may be some muscle development as a result of this type of training, but in most cases it's unlikely that this will be significant enough to have a negative impact on power-to-weight ratio by way of increased body weight. In fact, for many cyclists, some strengthening work can help improve lean muscle mass and enhance your fat-burning metabolism for a more athletic body.

The Essential Strength Exercises

Throughout this chapter I refer to movements more than to specific muscles. All the exercises here are compound functional movements where the whole body is working together to generate force. I will describe the main muscles involved but keep in mind that the movement is more important. For example, your squat strength is more important than your leg strength.

I will describe any specific cycling benefits first, then explain the relevance of each movement for day-to-day basic human fitness too, for injury prevention and for maintenance of musculoskeletal health.

The squat

For cyclists, the squat is an essential strength exercise for the quads at the front of the thigh, and the glutes and upper hamstrings at the back of the thigh and hips. These muscles are all prime movers on the pedalling downstroke and developing muscular strength here allows you greater potential for power production, particularly when kicking into an acceleration out of the saddle, such as when 'jumping' away from traffic lights or sprinting for a finishing line.

The squat forms the foundation for standing/sprinting power on the bike, as it is the foundational movement for any 'jump'. Squat work can be dovetailed with specific accelerations or 'jumps' to translate gains in strength to speed and power on the bike. Conditioning your body with a squat (and a bend too) while learning to maintain a neutral spine can also help you adopt this posture naturally and easily when confronted by day-to-day lifting and carrying tasks. This can prevent you incurring injuries off the bike that affect you on it.

The 'prime movers' are the main muscle driving any movement. Other muscles may be involved as helpers or stabilizers, but the prime mover is the one that generates force.

The squat is also essential because it targets some of the areas that tend to weaken because of the repetitive low-load nature of cycling and the limited range of the seated action. The medial or 'inner' portion of the quads, the upper hamstrings and glutes and the lower back are all areas that the squat develops in one movement. When performed with good form, the squat can begin to balance the load across these muscle groups to both improve performance and reduce the risk of knee injury in particular.

Because of the emphasis of the downstroke at low to moderate intensities, cyclists often become 'quad dominant', and the lateral or 'outer' part of the muscles in particular become overdeveloped, to the detriment of progressively weakening buttock muscles at the hips. With the medial (or 'inner') part of the quads being most active in the last 15 degrees of extension (leg straightening), the bent-knee seated cycling action can result in a relative weakness of one of the quad muscles called the vastus medialis (or VMO). This relative weakness is often implicated in knee pain and problems experienced by cyclists. Performing a full range squat while paying close attention to knee alignment can help correct this, particularly when coupled with pre-stretching the ITB with the foam roller exercise in Chapter 2.

If you have experienced knee problems associated with your cycling, I highly recommend you look to include some form of squat in your conditioning programme. Combining some squats with pre-stretches for the ITB in Chapter 2 and core strengthening exercises for the glutes in Chapter 4 may give you the best results.

The squats outlined in this section are described in progressive levels such that the more advanced version of the exercise comes at the end. If you have never used the squat as a strengthening exercise, progressing through each of the exercises in order will help you to learn correct form as you progressively add load.

Swiss ball supported squat

This version of the squat is an introductory exercise for those who have no experience of squatting, or want to learn the basics correctly before moving on. The support of the ball at the lower back makes it suitable if you know you have a weak back, or struggle with poor form and posture without any guidance. Using the ball helps to teach you how to maintain a neutral spine as you roll around it and down the wall, shifting your weight backwards at the same time as bending your knees. The curve of the ball supporting your lower back gives you direct feedback as you go through the movement because you can feel it if your back comes away from the ball.

Having the support of the ball can also help you focus on lifting your chest and engaging your abdominals by drawing your navel in, two important habits to establish to translate into safe loaded squatting.

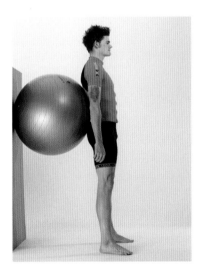

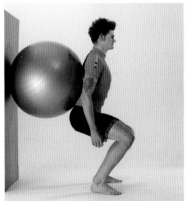

Preparation

Place the ball between you and the wall so that the curve of the ball supports the curve of your lower back. Your feet should be shoulder-width apart or slightly wider, with your feet turned out a little and slightly in front of your hips.

Movement

Roll down the ball into the squat or 'sit' position, ensuring you push back into the ball and roll around it so that no gap appears between you and the ball. As you do so, draw your navel in and lift your chest. Ensure that your knees track in line with your toes (and do not roll inwards or outwards). When learning the exercise, a brief pause at the bottom allows you to check this position. Then, push through your legs and buttocks to come up to the standing position.

How many reps and sets?

Perform 8–12 repetitions for 2–4 sets, with about 30 seconds between sets. At this stage the focus is on learning the movement and maintaining position and technique. If you want to add weight to this squat you can carry two dumbbells at your sides, in which case I recommend you increase the rest between sets to a minute. Once you feel you have exhausted the benefits from this variation, move on to one of the unsupported squats that follow.

The prisoner squat

A good body weight squat should be the foundation for any loading, and the 'prisoner squat' and 'stick' squats below form solid staples as general conditioning exercises, or as a warm-up before adding weight.

Both exercises teach correct alignment and balance while maintaining a neutral spine. The arm position in the prisoner squat and use of the stick in the stick squat help you engage the muscles of the upper back and shoulders. Some body weight squats can be performed without this emphasis (such as the 'arse-to-the-grass' primal squat mentioned in Chapter 1) but for the purposes of preparing to add weight to the bar or to carry it on the front of the body, these technique points are important.

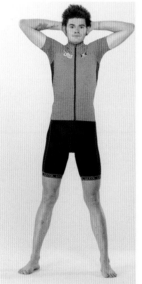
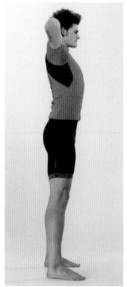
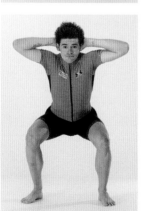
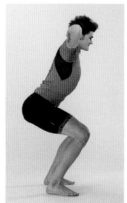

Preparation

Stand with your feet a little wider than shoulder-width apart, with your toes slightly turned out and your hands behind your head. Pull your elbows backwards, lift your chest and pull your shoulders down away from your ears.

Movement

Sit into the squat, as if you're sitting into a chair. Bend your knees and push your bum backwards. At the same time, open your elbows to the sides and lift your chest, pulling your shoulder blades together and down at the back. Keep your knees in line with your toes throughout. Go as low as you are able to maintain a neutral spine in your lower back and pause briefly at the bottom position before pushing up through the legs to stand up again. Try to keep your torso as upright as possible through the movement.

How many reps and sets?

Perform 8–12 repetitions for 2–4 sets, with 1 minute's rest between sets. At this stage the focus is on learning the movement and maintaining position and technique, particularly the extension through the upper back.

Stick squat

The most common way of loading a squat in the gym is with a barbell resting across the upper back. Practising with a stick can be useful in learning grip, stance and upper back engagement and position. Then when you start to use a squat rack you will know what to do once you have picked the weight up out of the rack. If you progress to using a rack, set the bar a little lower than shoulder height so that you 'sit' under the bar to pick it up.

Preparation

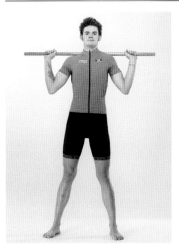 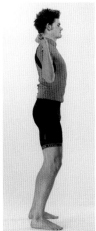

The stick should rest on the fleshy part of your upper back, not your neck. Grip the bar firmly just wider than shoulder width, squeeze your shoulder blades together and tuck your elbows under to engage your upper back to lift your chest.

Movement

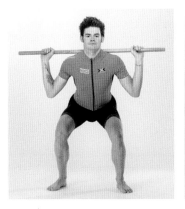 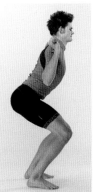

As you sit into the squat, keep tucking your elbows under, arch your lower back and lift your chest. Keep your knees in line with your toes. The weight should stay within your base of support. For example, a plumb line dropped from the end of the bar should fall through your foot.

How many reps and sets?

Perform 8–12 repetitions for 2–4 sets, with 1 minute's rest between sets. At this stage the focus is on learning the movement and maintaining position and technique, particularly the extension through the upper back and 'elbows under stick' position.

Overhead stick squat

The overhead squat is an excellent option with a stick or light bar if you want to progress but don't have access to heavier weights. This exercise is very demanding on your back, shoulders and core, but if you know you have a very stiff upper back it's probably not a good option for you as you will struggle to maintain good form. However, if you have good upper back mobility and no shoulder problems this exercise is a great variation.

Preparation

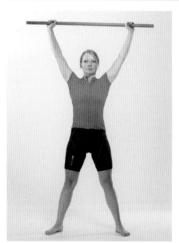 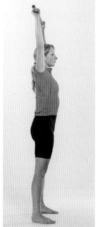

Using a similar grip width to the back squat, straighten your arms overhead, stretching your upper back as you do so, working hard so that the stick or light bar is directly overhead and not forwards of your body. It might help you to engage your upper back if you imagine pulling the two ends of the stick away from each other.

Movement

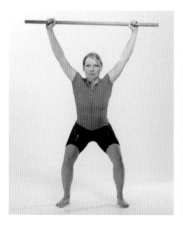 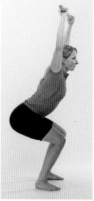

As you sit into the squat, keep extending your back and pulling backwards on your arms. Your goal is to keep the stick within your base of support (in line with your feet from the side as shown here). This type of squat works your trunk much harder than the other variations included here, so you will notice your back and abdominals really working hard, even without any weight.

How many reps and sets?

Perform 8–12 repetitions for 2–4 sets, with 1 minute's rest between sets. At this stage the focus is on learning the movement and maintaining position and technique, particularly the extension through the upper back.

Dumbbell front-loaded squat

The dumbbell front squat is the safest and easiest way to start to work with weight if you don't have access to a squat rack and bar. Holding the weight in front of your chest makes it easy and safe to load and lift a dumbbell into position without any special equipment like a squat rack.

Preparation

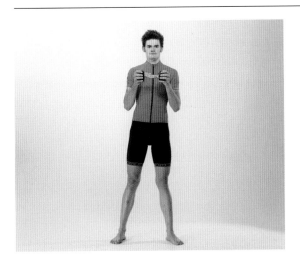

Hold the dumbbell in front of your chest as shown. Adopt a squat stance with your feet just outside your shoulders and turned out slightly.

Movement

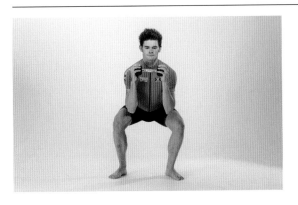

As you sit into the movement, bring your elbows forwards so that they stay under the dumbbell, not behind it. Lift your chest to work against the load so that it does not pull you forwards. Try to keep the weight of the dumbbell within your base of support (in line with your feet).

How many reps and sets?

Perform 8–12 repetitions for 2–4 sets, with 1 minute's rest in between sets. In practice, this means that you should be able to do between 8 and 12 repetitions of the exercise and you should be working hard to maintain your position and technique for the last two or three repetitions. Essentially, you should start to fail between 8 and 12 and should not be able to do more than 12, so if you find that you can you need to increase the weight of the dumbbell. If you are unable to do eight repetitions with good form with even a light weight, you can choose an easier version of the squat.

The dead lift (bend)

The dead lift is the most important conditioning exercise for cyclists to strengthen their back and hips. Learning correct movement technique in lifting and bending movements, and strengthening the muscles involved is vital if you want to prevent back problems getting in the way of your cycling. Strengthening your back and glutes by dead lifting will also provide more power to each pedal stroke when you ask for it, particularly when climbing, accelerating, or pushing hard while seated in the saddle.

The dead lift is the main back strengthening exercise you can include in your conditioning programme. Strengthening your back through this bending movement will help you to develop the robustness you need for long climbs, seated accelerations, or seated hard efforts along the flat. Dead lift work can be dovetailed with specific seated climbing intervals or accelerations to translate gains in strength to seated power on the bike.

The lower back is the most common problem area for cyclists and this is largely due to the poor posture associated with cycling, together with deconditioning in lifting and bending movements. The short and tight hamstrings and weakened core common among cyclists can change the postural curves of the spine, 'flattening' the lower back in particular by pulling down on the back of the pelvis.

This typical 'flat back' posture together with poor technique or awareness when bending forwards can lead to strains to the hamstrings and lower back muscles, as well as more serious injuries to the lumbar discs. For these reasons many cyclists avoid the dead lift movement for fear of injuring their back, but I would urge you to at the very least work towards including some dead lifting as part of your essential conditioning programme.

If you know you have a vulnerable back I would approach these dead lift exercises with care, but I would also urge you to make a point of making a start where you can. I have selected dead lift variations here that start with the very basics of body weight technique as an entry level exercise for everyone, even if you have back problems.

I have also described the movement from the 'top down' so that you can choose to work with a limited range if you are too tight in your hamstrings to lift a load off the floor with a neutral spine. Many cyclists will not be able to lift from the floor correctly to start with, but don't let this deter you from working with whatever range you have.

If you have a back problem associated with riding, combining these dead lifts with hamstring stretches from the essential stretches in Chapter 2 and the hip and back extensions from the core section in Chapter 4 will give you the best chance of progressing. Conditioning your body with a dead lift (and squat too) while learning to maintain a neutral spine can also help you adopt this posture naturally and easily when confronted by day-to-day lifting and carrying tasks. This can prevent you incurring injuries off the bike that affect you on it.

Short-stop position (dead lift preparation)

This short-stop position exercise is an entry level exercise to help you learn to move into the dead lift position correctly, and engage your core muscles in the way that you should to support your back. It is a body weight exercise, and unlike the other dead lift exercises it is more about developing the correct posture in the movement first, before looking to lift any weight. You will see this same exercise as preparation for the bent-over row too.

Preparation

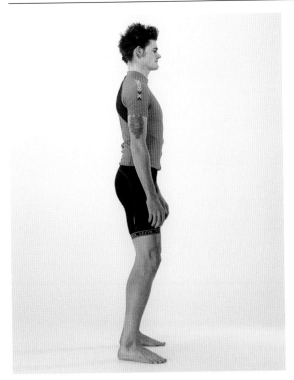

Stand with your feet shoulder-width apart or slightly wider, with your feet turned out a little. Lift your chest and lengthen your spine so that you are as tall as possible.

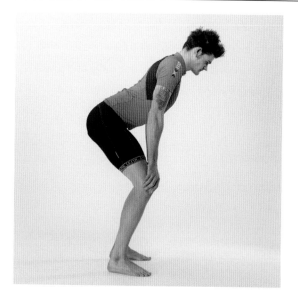

Resting your hands on your thighs, tip forwards from your hips so that you maintain a neutral spine, and at the same time bend your knees slightly. Keep tipping forwards in this way until your hands are just above your knees and your body is at a diagonal line as shown in the picture. Your thumb should be resting inside your knee and the rest of your fingers outside. Using a mirror to one side can be particularly helpful in checking that your body looks the way it should if you're not used to this kind of movement.

Once in this position, straighten your arms, pushing them into your legs so that you are actively using your upper body to brace yourself in the position. Draw your belly button back towards your spine so that you are engaging your deep abdominal muscle and hold the position. To come out of position, maintain the neutral spine in your back and the sensation of drawing in, and push through your feet and stand upright again, sliding your hands up your thighs as you go.

How many reps and sets?

This exercise is unlike all the other dead lift variations because you are looking to develop postural endurance in the position, rather than strength in the movement. It works well with progressively longer holds within each set. In the set descriptions below, 'on' means that you are in the position and 'off' means that you come out of the position.

3 × 20 seconds on 10 seconds off × 2–3 sets

3 × 30 seconds on 15 seconds off × 2 sets

3 × 45 seconds on, 15 seconds off × 2 sets

3 × 1 minute held with 30 seconds' rest × 1 set

Once you can effectively complete the final progression maintaining good form, you can be confident that you can progress to one of the lifting and moving dead lift variations that follow here.

Dumbbell dead lift

Preparation

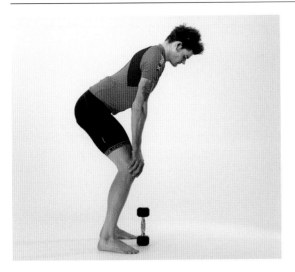

Place the dumbbell between your feet and adopt a shoulder-width stance either side of the weight. If you have a dumbbell with a flat end it might be easiest to rest it on that end, but if you are working with a spinlock dumbbell you will have to lay it on its side.

Tip forwards towards the weight using the 'short stop' technique from the previous exercise as shown below. Keeping the dumbbell close to your body is good practice, and if you are presented with an object that you need to lift, keeping it as close as possible will help you lift and move it more effectively.

Movement

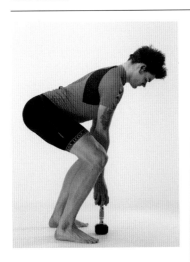
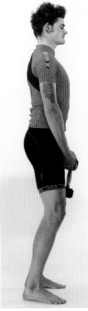

In order to reach the dumbbell and lift it off the floor, first arch your lower back as much as you can, as you tip forwards from the hips. Then bend your knees in a squatting action to reach the weight. As you bend towards the floor, keep your knees in line with your feet, and look down at the dumbbell.

Using your legs and back together, and engaging your abdominals by drawing your navel in, push with your feet and stand up tall with the dumbbell, keeping your back neutral. If you struggle to keep your back neutral to pick up the dumbbell from the floor, throughout the set work only within the range through which you can maintain an natural curve in the lower back, and then use your legs in a squatting action to place the dumbbell back on the floor at the end. With practice, and together with some stretching, you will find that you are able to increase your range of movement with good form.

Repeat this movement, tipping forwards from the hips towards the floor as far as you can maintain a neutral spine, and then pushing through your legs to stand up tall and straight. Your knees should always bend slightly to support your back throughout the movement, but not so much that the exercise becomes more of a squat than a bend.

Remember to distinguish between the squat and bend. In a squat the load is above your centre of gravity, while in a bend it is below. In the squat a knee bend initiates the movement and the torso stays relatively upright while in the bend a 'tipping' at the hips and back initiates the movement and the knees bend as a secondary motion.

How many reps and sets?

Perform 8–12 repetitions for two to four sets, with 1 minute's rest in between sets. In practice, this means that you should be able to do between 8 and 12 repetitions with good form and you should be working hard to maintain your position and technique for the last two or three repetitions. Essentially, you should start to fail between 8 and 12 and should not be able to do more than 12. If you find that you can, you need to increase the weight of the dumbbell. If you are unable to do 8 repetitions with good form with even a light weight, keep working on the short-stop exercise and come back to the dead lift later.

The split squat (lunge)

The split squat is an important exercise for cyclists for strengthening the legs and developing stability in the hips and muscles surrounding the pelvis. The narrow stance of the split squat can highlight any asymmetries in leg strength and pelvic stability and allow you to work towards better balance so that you are equally strong and stable on both sides, and avoid any problems that can result from a favoured or dominant side.

I have chosen to include the more static split squat here (instead of the more dynamic lunge) because its greater stability requirement is more relevant to cyclists, who need a stable pelvis to push from when both seated and standing on the bike. Dynamic forward lunges can tend to exacerbate the 'quad dominance' and relative weakness in the buttock muscles that is common and may provoke calf injuries in cyclists because of the eccentric 'braking' forces involved. This is another good reason to favour the split squat, back lunge or multidirectional lunge first, before introducing the forward lunge.

The split squat is an essential strength exercise for ensuring balance between the leg muscles and stability of the pelvis. Developing strength together with stability in the hips will help you to maintain a stable core as you generate force with your legs both in and out of the saddle.

For some cyclists who are stiff and tight in the hamstrings and weaker in the lower back, squats and dead lifts with a neutral spine may be difficult to work with, so the split squat offers a useful alternative leg-strengthening exercise as the torso stays upright throughout the exercise.

If you struggle with good form in the squat because of lack of flexibility in the hamstrings or poor posture, the split squat will allow you to strengthen your legs with good form more easily.

Stick supported split squat

Preparation

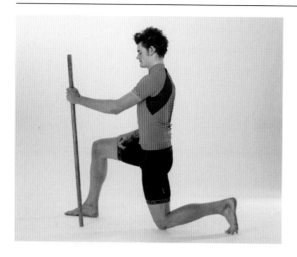

This supported split squat allows you to use a stick or empty light barbell to help to maintain good form and keep your body upright throughout the movement. The stick offers a support, making the split stance more stable if you struggle with the balance element. This variation will give you a feel for engaging your hip muscles on the back leg too, and help you avoid the problem of excessively leaning into the squat.

Start the movement from the bottom, so that you can check the width and length of your stance more easily Kneel in a split stance as shown, with both legs making a right angle at the knee. Your front shin and back thigh should be vertical, and your toes should be tucked under at the back, ready to push downwards.

Check that your feet are about hip-width apart, and that your back heel is aligned behind your buttock, and not turning inwards towards the middle of your body. This can be a common fault if you are tight in the hips and will make you unsteady when your push up into the split squat.

Movement

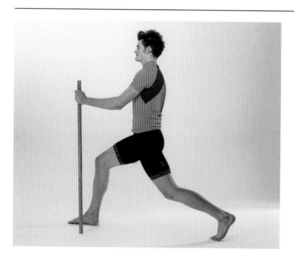

Tuck your hips down at the back and draw in your navel in to stabilize. Look forward, and keeping your body upright, push through both feet, and at the same time pull down on the stick to come up to the top of the split squat. Try to push through the ball of your foot on the back leg, kicking your heel up as you go. Your goal is to keep your spine 'neutral' and often this can mean quite a strong 'tuck' at the hips to engage the glute on your back leg.

Lower yourself with control back towards the floor, maintaining this position through the body until your back knee is hovering an inch or two away. Then, repeat the upwards push with both feet and pull downward on the stick to come back to the top position.

It's tempting at the top of the position to relax your body. Try to hold the tension in your torso so that you maintain a strong position throughout the exercise both on the up and the down of the movement.

How many reps and sets?

Perform 8–12 repetitions for 2–4 sets, with 1 minute's rest in between sets. For the split squat, one set means one set on each side. You should be able to do between 8 and 12 repetitions with good form, while working hard to maintain your position and technique for the last two or three repetitions. If you find that you are much better on one side than the other, only do as many reps as you can do well on your weakest side until you start to be able to work more evenly. For example, if you can only do 8 repetitions on your left side, you would only do 8 on your right side even if you could actually do more. You should start to fail between 8 and 12. If you find that you can do more than 12 repetitions well, you need to progress to one of the more difficult split squat options. If you are unable to do 8 repetitions with good form, keep working on the other exercises and come back to the split squat later.

Stick behind the head

This first unsupported split squat progression uses the stick across the upper back to help you engage your back and shoulder muscles, and to keep your torso engaged strongly throughout the movement. It will also help you keep your body upright and your core engaged, and avoid excessively leaning forwards. Using a stick across the back in this way also helps you to learn correct upper-body position for loading with a barbell later, if you decide to take your strengthening work into a gym.

Preparation

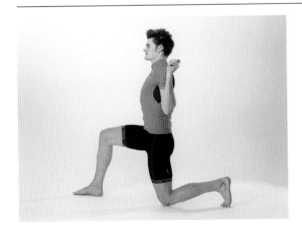

Starting from the bottom of the movement, so that you can check the width and length of your stance more easily, kneel in a split stance as shown with both legs making a right angle at the knee. Your front shin and back thigh should be vertical, and your toes should be tucked under at the back, ready to push downwards. Check that your back foot and front foot are about hip-width apart, and that your back heel is aligned behind your buttock, and not turning inwards towards the middle of your body. Make sure the stick is resting on the fleshy part of your upper back, not your neck, and lift your chest, squeeze your shoulder blades together, and tuck your elbows under the stick to engage the upper back muscles.

Movement

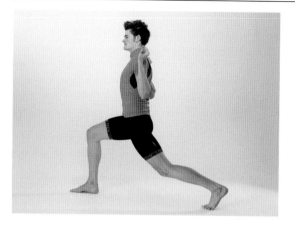

Prepare to push up into position by tucking your hips down at the back and drawing your navel in to stabilize your centre. Look forward, and keeping your body upright, push through both feet to come up to the top of the split squat. Try to push through the ball of your foot on the back leg, kicking the heel up as you go. Your goal is to keep your spine neutral, your chest lifted and your hips underneath your shoulders.

From the top position, lower yourself with control back towards the floor, maintaining this position through the body until your back knee is hovering an inch or two away. Then push with both legs to come back to the top position.

It's tempting at the top of the position to relax your body – your core and hips in particular. Try to hold the engagement in your torso so that you maintain a strong position throughout, both on the up and the down of the movement.

How many reps and sets?

Perform 8–12 repetitions for 2–4 sets, with 1 minute's rest in between sets. For the split squat, one set means one set on each side. You should be able to do between 8 and 12 repetitions with good form and you should be working hard to maintain your position and technique for the last two or three repetitions. If you find that you are much better on one side than the other, only do as many reps as you can do well on your weakest side until you start to be able to work more evenly. For example, if you can only do 8 repetitions on your left side, you would only do 8 on your right side even if you could actually do more. You should start to fail between 8 and 12. If you find that you can do more than 12 repetitions well, you need to progress to the dumbbell front-loaded option. If you are unable to do 8 repetitions with good form, keep working on the stick supported version until it becomes easier.

Dumbbell front-loaded split squat

This front-loaded split squat offers you a simple way to load the split squat for strength development without needing a gym. Make sure that you are able to perform the previous split squat variations well before progressing to this loaded option.

Preparation

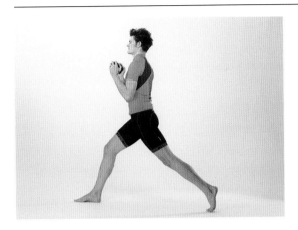

For this variation carrying a dumbbell, I recommend you start from the top of the movement. Hold the dumbbell in front of your chest with your elbows tucked directly underneath it. Actively use your upper back to keep your chest lifted to support the dumbbell in front of you.

To get into the correct position, start by standing with your feet hip-width apart, and then step into the split squat stance by taking two short strides forwards with whichever will be your front leg. Make sure your foot is straight, and not turned inwards or outwards. Check that your feet are hip-width apart and then kick up your back foot so that the weight is on the ball of your foot to prepare to move.

Movement

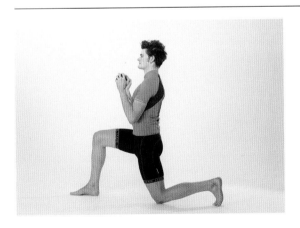

From the top position, shift downwards and slightly forwards with your hips, keeping the glute on the back leg engaged by tucking your pelvis down at the back and drawing your navel in to engage your abdominals. Keep your hips underneath your shoulders, and your chest lifted. Drop into the split squat by leading with your hips. Go low enough that your knee is about an inch or so off the ground. The knee may move slightly forwards of the ankle on the front leg throughout this movement. Then push through both legs, back up into the split stance position at the top of the movement. Repeat this movement at a steady speed without rushing, thinking about leading with your hips on the way down and your shoulders on the way up.

How many reps and sets?

Perform 8–12 repetitions for 2–4 sets, with 1 minute's rest in between sets. For the split squat, one set means one set on each side. You should be able to do between 8 and 12 repetitions with good form and you should be working hard to maintain your position and technique for the last two or three repetitions. If you find that you are much better on one side than the other, only do as many reps as you can do well on your weakest side until you start to be able to work more evenly. For example, if you can only do 8 repetitions on your left side, you would only do 8 on your right side even if you could actually do more. You should start to fail between 8 and 12. If you find that you can do more than 12 repetitions well, you need to progress by adding more weight to the dumbbell.

Pushing precautions

For cyclists, pushing movements should be carefully selected to ensure that strengthening occurs without exacerbating or contributing to poor posture. The 'prime movers' in pushing exercises are the chest muscles and the triceps at the back of the arm. Cyclists are often tight in the chest and stiff in the upper back with relatively shortened upper abdominal muscles pulling the ribcage down at the front to create a slumped position. These postural tendencies can make it difficult to maintain good alignment through a push, with the result often being excessive rounding of the upper back, so choosing an appropriate exercise for your current alignment is particularly important for pushing exercises.

Overhead pushing movements need to be approached with particular caution to avoid causing injury to the shoulder and/or neck in these circumstances. For cyclists who are rigid in the upper back with limited backwards bending (extension), overhead pushing and pressing movements can become risky or 'contraindicated'. When the upper back

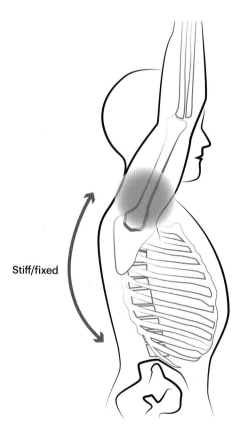

Stiff/fixed

Where some cyclists have a very stiff or 'fixed' thoracic spine, overhead loading may cause shoulder pain due to the disrupted biomechanics of the upper back and shoulder as they work together. If you failed the rib expansion test on page 53 or find the horizontal foam roller mobilization quite painful, you may want to avoid overhead pushing and pulling exercises until your back is more mobile

doesn't move adequately there is an increased likelihood of 'impingement' problems at the shoulder joint, in which case pushing movements that are forwards rather than upwards should be included until mobility is restored.

Shoulder impingement is a syndrome where the tendons of the rotator cuff muscles at the front of the shoulder become inflamed and irritated, leading to pain in the shoulder and arm, especially when raising your arm overhead or when lying on your side in bed at night. The space where the tendons exit the shoulder becomes reduced such that 'pinching' of the tendons occurs with certain movements. Impingement problems are more common with prolonged poor posture of the upper back, which can lead to bone changes in and around the shoulder joint.

'Contraindicated' is a medical term for something that is not advised. Certain exercises would be contraindicated for a particular person if they aggravate a condition or problem area. It's not that the exercise is 'bad', but that it's not a good idea for that person.

However, for those with already adequate mobility in the upper back, overhead pushes can be a good way to maintain flexibility and strengthen together. Single-arm pushes with a contralateral rotation (as with a punching action) are also an excellent way to include a push while keeping an eye on maintaining mobility.

Strictly speaking, the 'primal standard' for pushing exercises is one where you push and move a load forward while standing on your feet. For those who have access to a cable machine, single arm pushes with a twist can be a great way to maintain mobility while integrating the core and avoiding any unwanted upper body muscle development.

Without access to a cable machine and a gym, the pushing (and pulling) options are slightly limited. I have included two types of pushing exercises here, a closed-chain press-up and two open-chain options – the Swiss ball chest press and Swiss ball seated overhead shoulder press. Where possible, it's worth including both types of push as they each have their benefits. The closed-chain press-up requires more stability through the muscles of the upper back and shoulders, something that is also required when you hold the bars steady as you ride.

'Closed-chain' exercises are those where the hands (in an upper body exercise) are fixed and you move your body towards the unmoving surface. A press-up is an example of a closed-chain upper-body pushing exercise. An open-chain exercise is one where you move the load away from your body. The Swiss ball chest press here is an example of an open-chain pushing exercise.

Most functional exercises are closed chain in the lower body and open chain in the upper body. Force is generated from the ground up via the legs and transmitted through the core to be expressed through the arms. Squats, lunges and dead lifts are all closed-chain examples. The lunge-twist-push is an example of a closed-chain movement in the legs generating force that is expressed in an open-chain movement with the arm. Many functional movement combinations work in this way. For cyclists, seated cycling is an open-chain exercise and very sport specific. This is one of the reasons it's important to 'integrate' the strength you develop off the bike with goal-relevant interval training on the bike as part of your periodization.

The press-up (push)

The press-up is a long established classic core exercise combined with a body-weight push. Often used and rarely done well, a good press-up is an excellent exercise for abdominal strength, shoulder stability and pushing strength. The classic press-up also has the advantage of needing no equipment at all. A press-up performed with poor form can exacerbate poor posture and will do little to develop true strength in the body. Pay close attention to the 'form principle' here and choose the option that you can do well, or alternatively, if you struggle to maintain good alignment, choose the Swiss ball chest press instead and come back to the press-up later.

This press-up is the pushing option that strengthens the abdominal muscles the most, as well as developing shoulder stability. Being able to maintain neutral alignment of the spine is an essential prerequisite to including this exercise. If these are aspects you want to emphasize with your pushing choice, it will be a good option for you to include in your exercise programme.

Plank preparation

Most people fail to execute a good press-up because they have not developed a plank with good form first. This is why I have included a full plank as a preparatory exercise here. The press-up could quite legitimately be called a core exercise and therefore be included in Chapter 4, but since the pushing options for home-based exercise are limited, I have included it here.

Preparation

To prepare for a full plank position, start by kneeling with your knees and ankles together. Keeping the feet, ankles and knees together in the plank position can help you engage your hips when you push up into the plank position.

Kneeling plank position

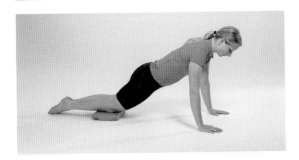

Keeping your hands a little wider than your shoulders, and with your fingers pointing forwards, walk your hands away from your knees and gradually drop your hips down, until you are in the position shown with your shoulders directly above your wrists and your knees, hips and shoulders in one line. In this position, focus on squeezing your glutes together, pulling your abdominals in, and keeping your shoulders down away from your ears.

For some (women in particular), this kneeling plank forms a good foundation for the kneeling press-up that will follow. Note that it is not a 'box' press-up. In this example, the trunk is in a straight line so that the core muscles are fully engaged.

Full plank position

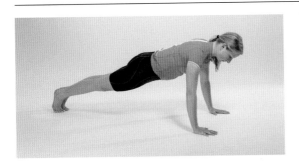

To push up into the full plank position from the kneeling plank, tuck your toes under and push back through the balls of your feet to lift the hips. The hips should not drop when you move into position but should actually lift slightly. Strengthen your middle by squeezing your glutes together and strongly bracing through the abdominals. Keep your arms straight and pull your shoulders away from your ears.

The plank position is one of those exercises that tests your ability to maintain a neutral spine. If you are holding good form, with a sense of working hard through your core, you are probably in a good position. If you are dipping into your lower back or rounding your upper back then you are not holding a good position and it might be best to leave this exercise out and keep coming back to it as you work on other areas to bring your body into better balance. Using a mirror to one side to make you more aware of your position can be really useful with this exercise.

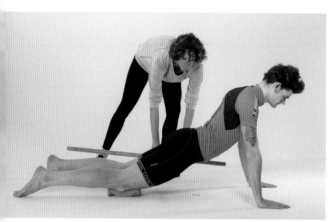

Here, Jake shows a classic pattern of a poor 'plank' position, with a dipped lower back and a rounded upper back. Even with me trying to correct and cue for the right position, Jake was unable to achieve good form at this stage in the exercise.

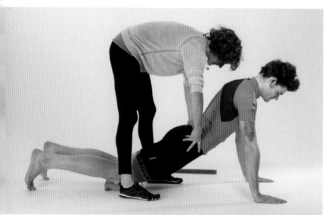

Kneeling press-up

Preparation

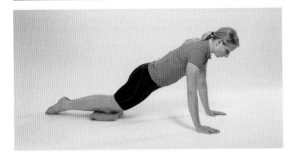

Adopt the kneeling plank position as described on page 127, with your hands positioned a little wider than your shoulders and your abdominals and glutes actively engaged.

Movement

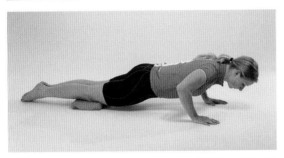

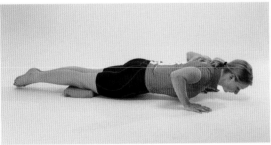

Lower your body directly to the floor with control, maintaining a straight line through your knees, hips and shoulders, until your hips and chest are touching the ground. Your elbows should move backwards slightly behind your shoulders as you move down and back up from the floor. Pause briefly as your hips touch the floor and then, pushing firmly with your arms and keeping your shoulders pulled down away from your ears, press up to the kneeling plank start position. Your hips and chest should come up off the floor at the same time if you are doing a good job of the press-up.

How many reps and sets?

Perform 8–12 repetitions for 2–4 sets, with 1 minute's rest in between sets. If you find you cannot do 8 repetitions with good form, just do as many as you can do well until you are able to do 8 in one set. You should be working hard to maintain your position and technique for the last two or three repetitions. If you find that you can do more than 12 good kneeling press-ups you should progress to the full press-up described on page 130.

Full press-up

Preparation

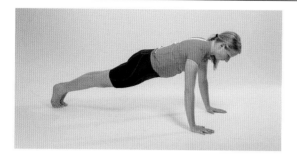

Adopt the full plank position as described on page 127, with your hands positioned a little wider than your shoulders and your abdominals and glutes actively engaged.

Movement

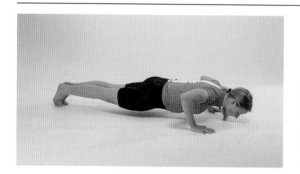

Lower your body directly to the floor with control, maintaining a straight line through your knees, hips and shoulders, until your hips and chest are hovering above the ground. Your elbows should move backwards slightly behind your shoulders as you move down and back up from the floor. Pause briefly as your hips reach the floor. Then push firmly with your arms, keeping your shoulders pulled down away from your ears, press up to the full plank start position. Your hips and chest should move at the same time if you are doing a good job of the press-up.

How many reps and sets?

Perform 8–12 repetitions for 2–4 sets, with 1 minute's rest in between sets. If you find you cannot do 8 repetitions with good form, just do as many full press-ups as you can do well and then complete the set by dropping to your knees for the kneeling press-up. You should be working hard to maintain your position and technique for the last two or three repetitions. If you find that you can do more than 12 good press-ups, you can progress the exercise by doing more repetitions or finding more challenging variations of the exercise. However, for most cyclists 10–12 good full press-ups is reasonable.

Swiss ball dumbbell chest press (push)

The Swiss ball chest press is an excellent option for cyclists, taking the more traditional bench press and moving it onto the ball for greater core engagement, and for ease of use at home without a bench. The bridge position that forms the basis for this pushing movement helps to strengthen the glutes, upper hamstrings and back, and the instability of the ball helps to stimulate and 'wake up' the core muscles while you are working at the push with your upper body. Getting into and out of position can take a bit of practice and it's important that you master this with only light (or no) load before adding significant weight to the exercise.

This chest press is a good option if you want to emphasize glute and back strength together with pushing strength. It is the safest option if you have a weak core and /or stiff upper back, and struggle with maintaining neutral alignment in the press-up. To ensure your back is safe, practise moving into and out of position first before adding load.

Preparation

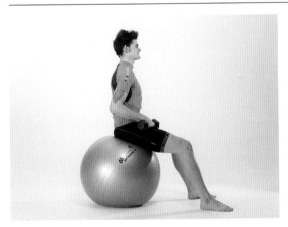

Hold your dumbbells at your hips while seated on the ball. From this seated position, walk your feet forwards and keep your weight over the ball until you are in a bridge position with your upper back and head supported by the ball, your chest and hips lifted, and your arms to the sides of your body. When moving into and out of position for this exercise, have faith in the ball and keep your weight firmly over it. The start position for the chest press is with the dumbbells held directly over your elbow as shown in the picture. Your knees should be over your ankles, and your knees, hips and shoulders should make one straight line to form your bridge foundation.

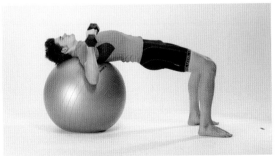

Movement

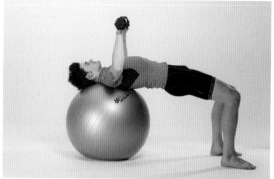

From this start position, push upwards against the dumbbells, bringing them together at the top of the movement in the centre of your chest, and then lowering them back to the start position by retracing the same pathway. The dumbbells should come up and together and then out and down in a smooth arc.

Keep your chest and hips lifted throughout the movement, with the dumbbells level with your chest (not your shoulders) and your shoulders pulled down away from your ears.

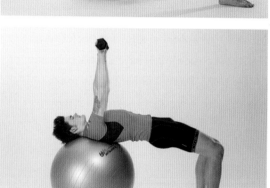

How many reps and sets?

Perform 8–12 repetitions for 2–4 sets, with 1 minute's rest in between sets. You should be able to do between 8 and 12 repetitions with good form and you should be working hard to maintain your position and technique for the last two or three repetitions. You should start to fail between 8 and 12. If you find that you can do more than 12 repetitions well, you need to progress by adding more weight to the dumbbells.

Swiss ball seated dumbbell shoulder press (push)

The seated shoulder press is a pushing option that emphasizes shoulder strength more than chest strength. As the dumbbells are pressed overhead, it also depends on good flexibility in the upper back in order to achieve good alignment and good form. In order to choose and include this pushing option, you should first ensure that your upper back extends (or bends backwards) well. Using the rib expansion test and the horizontal foam roller exercise from the essential stretching section in Chapter 2 will give you an idea of how flexible you are in this area. If you are unable to perform this exercise as described here, choose one of the other pushing options and come back to the shoulder press later.

If you already have good mobility in your upper back, this overhead press is an excellent option for maintaining flexibility in the upper back while at the same time developing pushing strength overhead. Sitting on the ball to perform the push also allows you to develop seated postural awareness and endurance.

Preparation

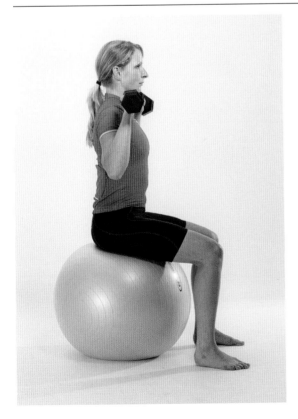

Start by sitting upright on the ball, with your feet a little wider than shoulder width and your knees in line with your ankles so that your lower leg is perpendicular. Lift the dumbbells to the start position so that they are just outside and slightly forwards of your shoulders, as shown here. When you look straight ahead you should just be able to see them in the corners of your eyes.

Movement

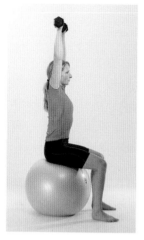 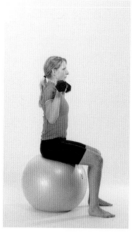

Keeping your chest lifted and your abdominals engaged, push the dumbbells directly upward, and then bring them together to touch overhead. To achieve this position you will need to extend your upper back by lifting your chest. From this top position, lower the dumbbells back to the start by retracing the same pathway they have just taken. The dumbbells should come up and together overhead, then out and down in a smooth arc, similar to that made with the dumbbell chest press.

How many reps and sets?

Perform 8–12 repetitions for 2–4 sets, with 1 minute's rest in between sets. You should be able to do between 8 and 12 repetitions with good form and you should be working hard to maintain your position and technique for the last two or three repetitions. You should start to fail between 8 and 12. If you find that you can do more than 12 repetitions well, you need to progress by adding more weight to the dumbbells.

The importance of pulling exercises

For those reasons explained earlier, my first choice of pulling exercises for cyclists would be cable machine exercises where pulling can be combined with squatting, lunging, twisting and bending movements to develop functional upper-body strength together with the legs. However, more 'isolated' pull variations that focus specifically on the upper-back muscles can be an important corrective and balancing exercise for cyclists who tend to have weak upper-back muscles together with poor posture and a stiff thoracic spine.

Often cyclists will experience neck problems on the bike when the biomechanics of their spine have been altered due to long-standing muscle imbalances and subsequent changes in the bone structure. Stiffness in the upper back transfers excessive strain to the neck, which must bend backwards more so the rider can look forwards at the road ahead.

Mobilizing the thoracic spine together with strengthening the upper back with pulling movements can help maintain a healthy upper back and neck, as well as improving the aesthetic and aerodynamic shape of the back on the bike that every cyclist is looking for.

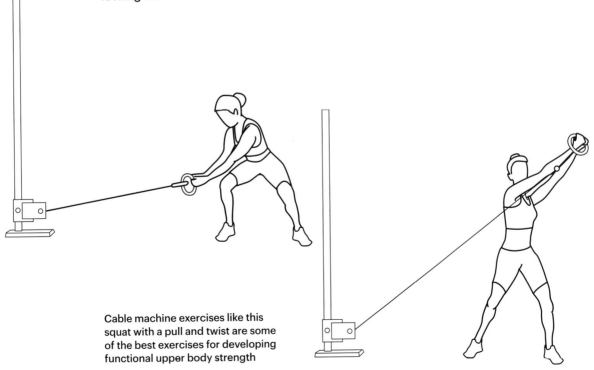

Cable machine exercises like this squat with a pull and twist are some of the best exercises for developing functional upper body strength

The bent-over row variations included here, performed with dumbbells, are a good example of somewhat 'isolated' pulling exercises that develop the strength of the upper back together with enhancing postural endurance of the lower back by holding the position. The 'prone cobra' exercise included in Chapter 4 is even more isolated still, forcing extension of the upper back by lifting the chest off the floor.

Taken together, the prone cobra and these rowing exercises are the most important exercises you can include for strengthening the upper back to improve your cycling position or 'flat back' posture, as well as to prevent neck problems.

In terms of cycling performance, in a seated climb where the load is heavy and the pedalling cadence is slow, there should be a natural pulling action on the arm on the same side as the downwards pushing leg. This 'stabilizing' force assists by avoiding any movement at the bars while generating as much power as possible through the legs. As the force increases further and the power demands go beyond what is possible seated, when you stand out of the saddle the pulling action through the arms contributes more dynamically to the power and ground speed, moving the bike laterally from left to right and adding precision and power to the 'stepping' action on the pedal.

Pulling exercises are not only important for your posture both on and off the bike, but will also help you develop the strength you need in your upper body for improved efficiency when climbing seated in the saddle under heavier load, and in particular when you stand up out of the saddle. Pulling strength is also an important element of sprinting technique, allowing you the strength you need to develop an arm action that complements your leg speed and power.

The bent-over row (pull)

The bent-over row is an essential strengthening exercise that actually ticks two primal pattern boxes in one go, strengthening the upper back with a pulling movement, while strengthening the lower back as you hold the 'bend'.

You will see some overlap here with the instructions for the dead lift earlier and in fact the first technique drill is exactly the same for both. As always, correct alignment is important in order for the exercise to have maximum impact, so it is worth taking your time to work through the progressions here, starting with getting the basic position right before you add any weight.

Short-stop position (bent-over row preparation)

This short-stop position exercise is an entry level exercise to help you learn to move into the dead-lift position correctly and engage your core muscles in the way that you should to support your back. It is a body weight exercise, and unlike the other dead-lift exercises it is more about developing the correct posture in the movement first, before looking to lift any weight. You will see this same exercise as preparation for the bent-over row too.

Preparation

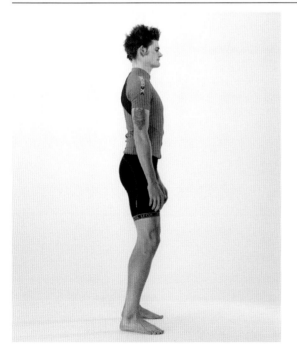

Stand with your feet shoulder-width apart or slightly wider, with your feet turned out a little. Lift your chest and lengthen your spine so that you are as tall as possible.

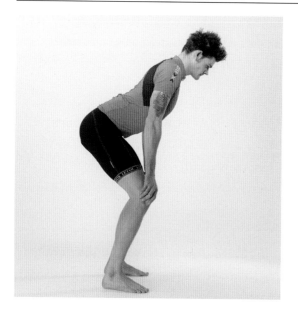

Resting your hands on your thighs, tip forwards from your hips so that you maintain a neutral spine, and at the same time bend your knees slightly. Keep tipping forwards in this way until your hands are just above your knees and your body is in a diagonal, as shown in the picture. Your thumb should be resting inside your knee and the rest of your fingers outside. Using a mirror to one side can be particularly helpful in checking that your body looks the way it should if you're not used to this kind of movement.

Once in this position, straighten your arms, pushing them into your legs so that you are actively using your upper body to brace yourself in the position. Draw your navel in so that you are engaging your deep abdominal muscles, and hold the position. To come out of position, maintain the neutral spine in your back and the sensation of drawing in, and push through your feet and stand upright again, sliding your hands up your thighs as you go.

How many reps and sets?

This exercise is unlike all the other dead lift variations because you are looking to develop postural endurance in the position, rather than strength in the movement. It works well with progressively longer holds within each set, and 1–2 sets of each progression is enough. In the set descriptions below, 'on' means that you are in the position, and 'off' means that you come out of the position.

10 seconds on, 10 seconds off × 6

20 seconds on, 10 seconds off × 3

30 seconds on, 15 seconds off × 3

45 seconds on, 15 seconds off × 3

Once you can effectively complete the final progression maintaining good form, you can be confident that you can progress to one of the lifting and moving dead lift variations that follow here.

Dumbbell bent-over row

Preparation

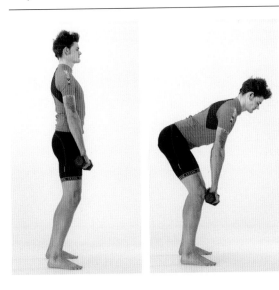

Stand tall with good posture with the dumbbells resting on your upper thighs. From here, tip forwards from the hips, lengthening your lower back and bending your knees slightly. As you tip forward, allow the dumbbells to slide down your thighs until they are hanging just above and slightly forwards of your knee.

Movement

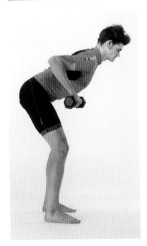
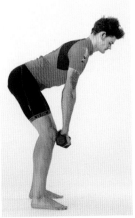

From this hanging position, pull the dumbbells upwards and into your body in a rowing action, leading with your elbows so that they come out and wide of your body. At the end of the pulling movement, make sure that your shoulder blades squeeze together. For this exercise I recommend a brief pause in this 'squeeze' position to emphasize the work in the mid-back muscles and make sure your neck is relaxed. Then, lower the dumbbells back to the start position, retracing the vertical line that they followed on the way up.

How many reps and sets?

Perform 8–12 repetitions for 2–4 sets, with 1 minute's rest in between sets. You should be able to do between 8 and 12 repetitions with good form and you should be working hard to maintain your position and technique for the last two or three repetitions. You should start to fail between 8 and 12. If you find that you can do more than 12 repetitions well, you need to progress by adding more weight to the dumbbells.

Swiss ball prone row

This Swiss ball prone row is a good variation if you struggle with the position and alignment of the 'bend' part of the bent-over row, allowing you to work the muscles of the upper back (and lower back) without needing to hold the sometimes difficult bent-over position. It's more isolated than the standing bent-over row and therefore is a crossover exercise between strength and core.

Here I am working with Jake to get him in a good short-stop/bent-over row/dead-lift position. For some cyclists, this will remain a struggle without anyone helping you to get the position right. If you have tried to get into position for the dead lift and bent-over row, and struggled, this next exercise is a good option for you to try.

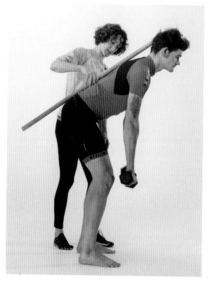 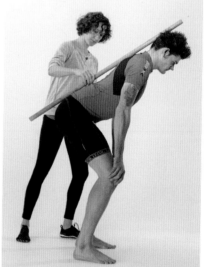

Preparation

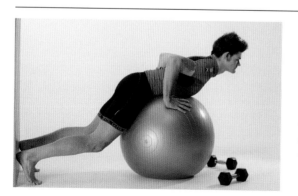

For this exercise you need to rest your feet against a wall or solid piece of furniture. Lying over the ball on your front, position your feet wide against the wall so that the balls of your feet are in contact with the ground and your heels are up the wall. Position the ball so that it's underneath your hips and pelvis, not too far forwards or back. You should place the dumbbells slightly in front of the ball and to the sides, so that you can reach them easily as you prepare for the rowing movement.

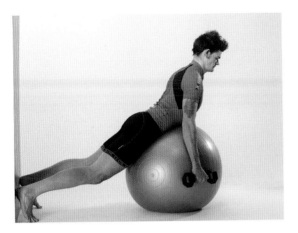

Next, take hold of the dumbbells and push your hips firmly into the ball, thrusting your hips forwards and tucking your tail bone down at the back. Actively engage your core as you then lift your upper back off the ball into the ready position.

Movement

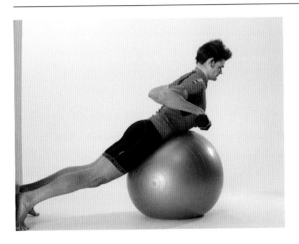

Maintaining the extended position throughout the rowing exercise, pull the dumbbells upwards and outwards in a rowing action, leading with your elbows so that they come out and wide of the ball. At the end of the pulling movement, make sure that your shoulder blades squeeze together. For this exercise I recommend a brief pause in this 'squeeze' position to emphasize the work in the mid-back muscles. Then, lower the dumbbells back to the start position, retracing the line that they followed on the way up. It's important with this variation that you keep your body still as you move your arms in the rowing action. You may find that your legs and back are working quite hard just to hold the position, but this is part of the exercise, so persevere and you will find you get stronger.

How many reps and sets?

Perform 8–12 repetitions for 2–4 sets, with 1 minute's rest in between sets, relaxing forwards over the ball. You should be able to do between 8 and 12 repetitions with good form and you should be working hard to maintain your position and technique for the last two or three repetitions. You should start to fail between 8 and 12. If you find that you can do more than 12 repetitions well, you need to progress by adding more weight to the dumbbells.

Twisting options

The classic standing twisting movements are variations of the 'chop', in which the prime movers are the abdominal obliques that rotate the core, together with the associated 'anterior sling' muscles from the adductor of the inner thigh, to the opposite shoulder. In the 'reverse chop' (its opposing movement), the prime movers are those that rotate the core from behind – the 'posterior sling' from the glute on the driving leg to the opposite latissimus dorsi.

To fully develop your twisting strength you will need to include movements outside the scope of what is possible with a simple set of dumbbells and a Swiss ball at home. If you have an athletic background and have exhausted the options here, it might be worth speaking to a personal trainer or strength and conditioning coach who can suggest some more dynamic standing twisting variations for you to include as part of your training programme.

Working at home with just a ball and dumbbells makes it harder to include some strengthening twists in your programme, but the ones I have included here offer an introduction to ensure you maintain the mobility of the spine needed for effective rotational strength in the back and abdominal muscles, and without becoming 'flexion dominant', which is a risk for cyclists who rely on many cross-crunch type exercise variations for their twist strength.

The movements I have included here are somewhat isolated because of the limitations created by working with just the basics at home. As a result you will see that there is some crossover between the exercises here and the core essentials in Chapter 4. For example, I have included an upper-body Russian twist here in the essential strength chapter, while there is a lower-body Russian twist in the core chapter.

In practice, using a mixture of the twisting exercises included here together with the more isolated core variations in Chapter 4 will keep you mobile and strong enough in the upper body, helping to improve your cycling posture and optimize your bike fit. Mobility together with improved strength in the upper back can also help prevent neck problems.

Swiss ball seated reverse wood chop (twist)

This dumbbell exercise targets the muscles of the upper back while encouraging mobility in the same area. I have chosen to include this exercise seated on the ball because for most cyclists it will be easier to maintain good form in a seated position than when standing, and it will help you target the exercise to the upper back where your body needs the work the most.

Preparation

Start by sitting upright on the ball, with your feet a little wider than shoulder width and your knees in line with your ankles so that your lower leg is perpendicular. Grasp one dumbbell with both hands, the underneath hand being the dominant one (the one in the direction of the movement), and the other hand wrapping over the top for support. If you are rotating to the left, your left hand is the dominant hand, if you are rotating right, your right hand is dominant.

Movement

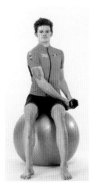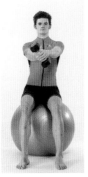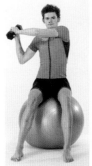

Keep your head facing forwards as your torso rotates and, drawing a diagonal line across your body, pull with your dominant hand, keeping your arms straight through the midpoint of the movement (shown centre) until the dumbbell is level with the opposite shoulder (shown right). Then, retrace the movement in reverse, following the same line as you return to the start position shown. As you move the dumbbell, try to keep your hips still and rotate through your torso, lifting your chest as you raise the dumbbell.

How many reps and sets?

Perform 8–12 repetitions for 2–4 sets, with 1 minute's rest in between sets. For this exercise you can do both sides together for one set, and then take the minute's rest, before doing both sides again. You should be able to do between 8 and 12 repetitions with good form and you should be working hard to maintain your position and technique for the last two or three repetitions. If you find that you are much better on one side than the other, only do as many reps as you can do well on your weakest side until you start to be able to work more evenly. For example, if you can only do 8 repetitions on your left side, you would only do 8 on your right side even if you could actually do more. You should start to fail between 8 and 12. If you find that you can do more than 12 repetitions well, you need to progress by adding more weight to the dumbbell.

Swiss ball cross crunch/chop (twist and bend)

This Swiss ball chop uses gravity together with the supine position to work the abdominal muscles in a twisting and chopping movement. This exercise is a good option for you if you already have good upper-back mobility as you bend and extend over the ball, but should be approached with caution if you are stiff in the thoracic spine.

To test whether this exercise is a suitable option for you, perform the rib expansion test as outlined in Chapter 2 on essential stretching and work into the exercise with caution, increasing the range of movement progressively by working in a more extended (backwards) position as you get used to it. If you know you have a rigid upper back or experience neck problems, or have difficulty looking up overhead, then this may not be a good choice of exercise for you.

Preparation

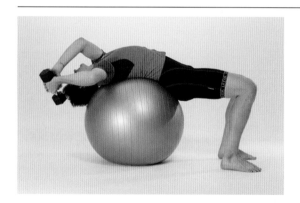

From a seated position, and keeping the dumbbell over your hips as you roll, shift your weight forwards down the ball and lie backwards over it until your back is arched over the ball with your hips and head both resting on the ball. Notice that the ball supports the spine along its length and your hips are resting on the ball (rather than lifted as in the bridge position needed for the chest press described earlier).

Grasp the dumbbell with the hand on the side to which you are going to pull the weight, and wrap your other hand around it for support. In the picture here Jake is chopping to the left, so his left hand is the dominant hand and his right hand is wrapped around for support. Reaching up and overhead with both hands, take the dumbbell above the opposite shoulder, so that you are being stretched backwards and diagonally against the load of the weight.

Movement

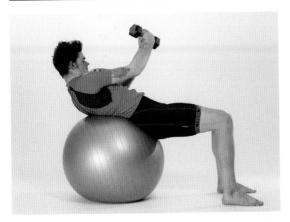

From this position, pull the weight over your head and diagonally towards the opposite hip, tucking your hips under so that your hips come up to meet the weight as it comes down. Briefly, hold his end position and engage your abdominal muscles fully before releasing back by retracing the pathway taken by the dumbbell to return to the start position.

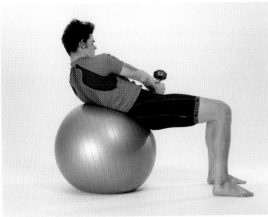

How many reps and sets?

Perform 8–12 repetitions for 2–4 sets, with 1 minute's rest in between sets. You should be able to do between 8 and 12 repetitions with good form and you should be working hard to maintain your position and technique for the last two or three repetitions. You should start to fail between 8 and 12. If you find that you are much better on one side than the other,

only do as many reps as you can do well on your weakest side until you are able to work more evenly. For example, if you can only do 8 repetitions on your left side, you would only do 8 on your right side even if you could actually do more. If you find that you can do more than 12 repetitions well, you need to progress by adding more weight to the dumbbells.

Swiss ball upper body Russian twist (twist)

Using the supine bridge position on the ball coupled with an upper-body twist, this exercise focuses the rotation on the upper back where cyclists can tend to be stiff and immobile. There is a balance element to this exercise and you will need to be quite confident moving into and out of position on the ball without falling off, so be alert!

In addition to working the upper back, the bridge position has the advantage of strengthening the hips and back at the same time.

Preparation

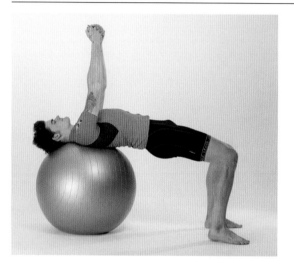

From a seated position on the ball, walk your feet forwards and keep your weight over the ball until you are in a bridge position with your upper back and head supported by the ball, your chest and hips lifted, and your arms extended, palms together as shown. When moving into and out of position for this exercise the trick is to trust the ball and keep your weight firmly over it. Your knees should be over your ankles, and your knees, hips and shoulders should make one straight line to form your bridge foundation.

Movement

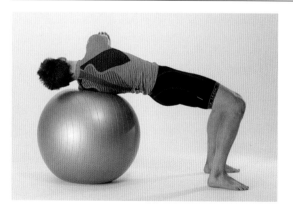

Keeping your hips lifted throughout, pull on your shoulder and turn your upper body in that same direction, focusing your effort on getting the ball moving underneath you. Your arms should stay straight and solid, imagining them as an extension of your upper body and torso.

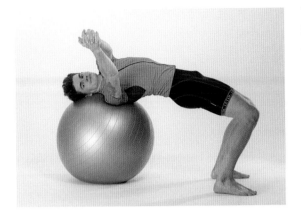

When you cannot rotate any further, pull back to the centre position and re-establish your position and balance, before pulling with the shoulder on the other side to twist in the opposite direction.

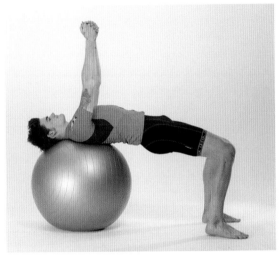

When you first learn this exercise it's best to stop in the centre position between each rotation, but as your balance improves and you become more dynamic on the ball you will be able to move straight through the centre position to turn to the other side.

How many reps and sets?

Perform 8–12 repetitions for 2–4 sets, with 1 minute's rest in between sets. For this exercise 8–12 repetitions represents the total number of reps on alternating sides. You should be able to do between 8 and 12 repetitions with good form and you should be working hard to maintain your position and technique for the last two or three repetitions. You should start to fail between 8 and 12. If you find that you can do more than 12 repetitions well, you need to progress by holding a dumbbell in both hands (wrapping one around the other, as with the previous reverse chop exercise) which significantly increases the challenge of the exercise.

Essential strength
ready reference pictures

The squat

Swiss ball supported

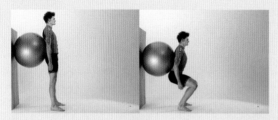

Prisoner squat/stick squat

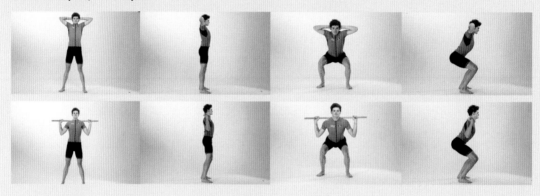

Overhead stick squat

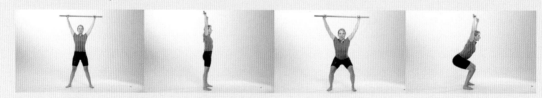

Dumbbell front loaded squat

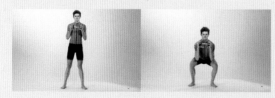

Dead lift

Short-stop position

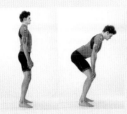

Dumbbell dead lift

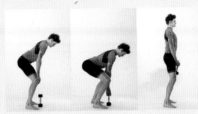

Split squat

Supported

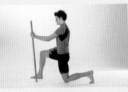

Behind the head

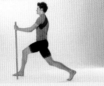 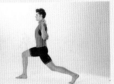

Dumbbell front-loaded split squat

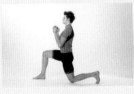 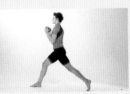

Press-up

Plank preparation (pics repeated with press-ups)

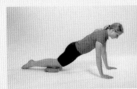 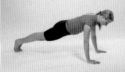

Kneeling press-up

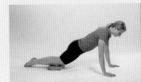 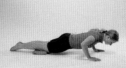 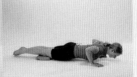

Full press-up

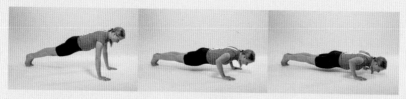

Swiss ball dumbbell chest press

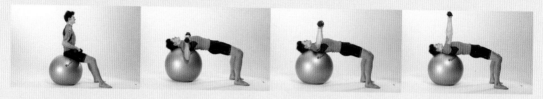

Swiss ball shoulder press

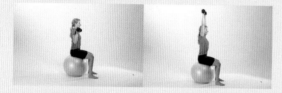

Bent-over row

Short-stop preparation
(repeated exactly as for the dead lift)

Dumbbell

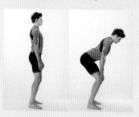

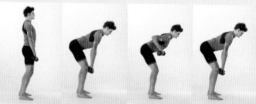

Swiss ball row

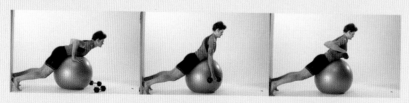

Swiss ball seated reverse wood chop

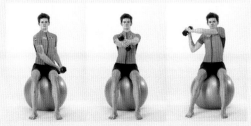

Swiss ball cross/crunch (chop)

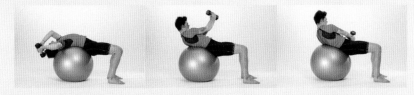

Swiss ball upper body Russian twist

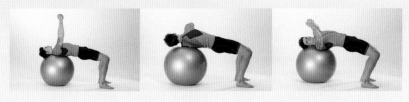

4. Essential core

What is 'core'?

The term 'core' has largely been popularized in the fitness industry to describe exercises that target the mid-section of the body, for the most part the abdominal muscles. Among sports coaches and strength and conditioning professionals in particular there is a different approach taken to the terminology; the word 'core' will be frowned upon, and instead 'the trunk' will be the favoured descriptor for the midsection, including your hip, abdominal and back muscles.

There is a certain amount of snobbery around this distinction, at the root of which is the understanding that there is no such thing as a core muscle, since all the muscles of the body work in interrelated chains, and those that cross the pelvis and spine in particular can have multiple roles in stabilizing or moving depending on the movement being executed. Any muscle that has an influence on the spine and pelvis could be called a core muscle, which leaves very few muscles that aren't technically core muscles at the edges of your body, like those of your arms and legs. The more fitness-orientated term 'core' has also been used as a marketing tool to capture the attention of people looking for a flat stomach and an aesthetic look, while the term 'trunk' acknowledges the role of the midsection in a more functional way, connecting the upper and lower body, the front and back of the body, and the left and right of the body.

In this book I am using the term 'core' to describe the mid-section of the body, both in terms of the muscles involved – including the hips, back and abdominals – and in terms of their function in keeping you injury free and performing at your best. It is outside the scope of this book to describe in great detail the anatomical function of each of the muscles, as I'm more concerned with giving you a broader understanding of what to do to effectively balance your core to become a stronger rider.

Why do cyclists need core training?

Core training has become a catch-all buzzword for something we should all be doing, cyclists included. But not only is there confusion around what the term means, but also around how you should train your core to prevent injury and maximize performance. 'Core weakness' is a blanket reason given for injury too, to the lower back and knees in particular, but there can be many different dimensions to a 'weak' core that lead to injury and limit performance. Usually where some muscles are weak, others have become tight. I have explained in some depth those muscles that tend to become tight in Chapter 2, so in this chapter I am turning my attention to those muscles that tend to become weak. Both stretching the tight *and* strengthening the weak will give you the best chance of bringing your core into balance.

The approach I am taking here is to illustrate some essential core exercises that target and strengthen the core muscles that tend to become weak in cyclists. The exercises will help you to coordinate and engage the 'inner' and 'outer' muscles of your abdomen, appropriately strengthen your hips and back, and learn correct alignment and posture to support your spine. The goal is to restore and maintain normal length-tension relationships in the muscles around joints to maximize cycling performance and reduce risk of injury.

The core exercises here will target the muscle areas that tend to weaken because of the cycling position, and also those that weaken due to the repetitive pedalling action. They will also take into account that the cycling position together with a desk job can lead to poor posture, increasing risk of injury and poor performance. The core essentials I have included here are easy to do effectively and target specific isolated areas to bring your body into balance.

Many forms of exercise incorporate elements of core work. However, some of the movements and exercises involved may be quite complex and seem difficult to follow or understand, so using the exercises here as a foundation will be most useful to start with.

The cross-training options that might enhance your core strength and control further will be discussed later in Chapter 5 on 'cross-training'.

Many core exercises can be a poor choice for cyclists because they tend to emphasize flexion (such as in any variation of a sit-up). And others can be too challenging for a cyclist's body that is too deconditioned at the outset to achieve good form (a plank can be another example here). Since cyclists often have poor posture with rounded shoulders and a flattened lower back, some of these exercises can actually make the balance and alignment of the muscles around the core worse, leading to an increased risk of injury. Poor posture and alignment is a sign of core weakness in itself, indicating that some tight muscles (or joints) are pulling the body out of position while others are unable to hold the body still. A cyclist's deeper core muscles (those responsible for postural endurance and maintaining a stable spine) are often weak and relatively 'switched off' too, which makes many of the more challenging core exercises out in general circulation relatively high risk for cyclists who have never done any conditioning off the bike before.

Consequently, you need to be discerning about your choice of core exercise to ensure that your intention to improve your core strength is matched by your exercise selection. Exercises that strengthen the core without flexion ('crunching') would be my favoured abdominal exercise options for cyclists, together with back strengthening exercises that encourage extension (or backwards bending) because they can help to correct for the slumped posture that often comes with bike riding and sitting at a desk. The essential core exercises included here will strengthen your core while bringing your body as a whole into better alignment. Exercises that emphasize the deeper muscles of the core are also included. These exercises are often missed out because they are more difficult to execute well and sometimes it's hard to feel like you are doing anything at all. In this chapter you will find core exercises that challenge you in three dimensions, another important facet in a well-balanced core programme.

The essential core exercises in this chapter are somewhat isolated, targeting several key muscle areas at a time in a focused way, working the deeper and more superficial muscles in three dimensions. They have been chosen because they help to correct for the postural tendencies of cyclists, bringing your body into better alignment while at the same time strengthening weakened muscles for injury prevention and optimal performance. They have also been chosen because I believe you will be able to do them effectively without any assistance from an exercise professional.

 # Problems associated with a weak core and the benefits of focused work

Most cyclists will be unaware they have a weakness in their core until they experience an injury. In practice, many injuries result from a combination of weak muscles and corresponding tight muscles, and often both need to be addressed to get to the root of the problem. For some riders, tightness may be an issue more than weakness, and for others it will be vice versa, but it's likely both will be implicated.

Often injuries are the result of both problems collaborating together. For example, lower back pain caused by lifting something is often caused by a combination of short and tight hamstrings pulling on the back of the pelvis together with weakened abdominal muscles that fail to engage properly upon bending forwards. The tight hamstrings and weak abdominal muscles together alter the biomechanics of the bend movement, leading to injury.

Cycling-specific issues that relate to the same imbalance would include lower back pain when pushing harder, such as when climbing in the saddle or pushing hard on the flats. This would be particularly noticeable if the saddle is set slightly too high, where the pull of tight hamstrings will cause excessive flattening of the lower back, coupled with the abdominal muscles being unable to stabilize the spine against the increased load. Lifting injuries and lower back pain on the bike both have at their root a muscle imbalance that leads to injury.

'Instability' is a term sometimes used in connection with your core to describe an erratic pattern of problems. For some people, a core weakness will manifest itself in a consistent injury or type of injury that recurs as a result of a similar movement or type of training. Others may experience a number of injuries with seemingly varied causes and symptoms that move around and seem unconnected, but at their root have a weak core.

It's common for a weak core to inhibit your progress only when you start to push yourself harder, either by doing some conditioning work off the bike or by having a more focused approach to your cycling training. A sudden increase in the intensity of exercise, such as when introducing hill repeats or sprints, or by launching into some weight training without adequate preparation, will likely lead to discomfort, pain or simply poor performance as a result.

The harder you push on the pedals with your legs (and pull with your arms, particularly when out of the saddle), the stronger your core needs to be to stabilize against the force you are generating. A stable and strong core will transfer these forces through your centre to the pedals without any problems. A weak core will cause a change in your cycling position at the hips and sometimes the knees too, causing an increased likelihood of pain and injury here.

Cyclists who go to the mountains of Europe for a cycling holiday for the first time may experience these core-related problems, as will those who take part in hilly sportives or harder races without adequate progression in training. Suddenly your back aches on the bike, and sometimes off it too, when you otherwise have been able to cycle for hours at your own pace without any problems. These issues may seem to come out of the blue but in fact the underlying weakness has been there all along, unchallenged by the type of riding that you are doing.

Symptoms of a weak core

- Recurrent pain or injury to your back or knees in particular
- Increased pain and problems with harder efforts such as hills and sprints
- Increased pain and problems with longer rides
- Poor posture, technique and style at higher intensities in particular (as indicated by nodding, shoving or rocking and rolling in the saddle)
- Poor performance at higher intensities – such as lack of power on the flats or uphill
- Increased risk of injury off the bike, particularly when lifting, carrying and moving heavy objects

Benefits associated with strengthening your core

- No pain or problems at higher intensities or for longer durations
- A sense of solidity through your core when pushing harder on the pedals
- Good posture, technique and style on the bike at all intensities
- Improved potential for optimal performance with hard training

Remembering the success formula

If you recognize your own pattern of injury and issues in the discussion here, or have not done any conditioning off the bike before, you will definitely benefit from 3–6 months of focused work on the exercises in this section. If you are not sure if your problems are caused predominantly by tightness or core weakness, then take the essential stretches from Chapter 2 that you found the hardest and use them in conjunction with some of the core exercises here. I will explain how to combine the various elements of essential conditioning for maximum effect in Chapter 6 on periodization and programme design.

If you found that in working through the essential stretches in Chapter 2 you seemed fairly flexible, a focused core programme may be the best place to start with your conditioning plan. For a small minority of cyclists (more often women), hypermobility can be the cause of recurrent injuries, issues and poor performance. If you know that you have tendencies towards hypermobility, including some of the core exercises in this chapter all year round will help you avoid any of the associated problems. The more hypermobile you are, the more stable you need to become to avoid injury and to maximize your performance.

'Hypermobility' or 'hypermobility syndrome' is a term given to people whose joints are inherently 'loose' or unstable. People who tend towards hypermobility often seem quite flexible in their muscles, but don't necessarily have the inherent normal level of stiffness in their joints to protect them from injury. Laxity or looseness in the connective tissue of joints can make you vulnerable to ligament sprains, minor joint subluxations (where a joint is pulled slightly out of alignment) and even complete dislocations of joints (for example, in the shoulders). If you are hypermobile you will do well with an essential conditioning programme that includes some of the essential core exercises here together with some more integrated strength exercises from Chapter 3 as you develop your programme year on year.

Remember the success formula:

FLEXIBILITY
+ CORE STABILITY
+ STRENGTH
= **POWER POTENTIAL**

Remember the success formula dictates that you prioritize each stage progressively in order to maximize your progress, so if you have a weak core, you will do well to focus on the essential core exercises here before introducing some more integrated strength work by adding some of the essential strength exercises in Chapter 3.

Weakness caused by the cycling position – the upper and lower back

The cycling position itself is one of the main reasons for core weakness. Physically we are designed to function upright, so prolonged periods spent bent over the bike can lead to some muscles becoming weak. Compared to our upright biomechanical norm, the forwards bend of the body on the bike can weaken the muscles of the lower back, those along the length of the spine and across the shoulder blades. Sitting in the saddle and bending forwards to reach the bars for hours at a time, the muscles along the back of the body are in a lengthened position and are relatively inactive at the low to moderate intensities which are typical for the bulk of a cyclist's training.

The cycling position itself can lead to weak core muscles if no balancing movements are included in a conditioning programme to help correct for the position. Some of the essential core exercises in this section focus on strengthening the back muscles that can become weak because of the cycling position. These include the muscles of the lower and upper back, as well as the muscles across the mid-back between the shoulder blades.

Weakness caused by the cycling action – the gluteals and upper hamstrings

The movement limitations of the pedalling action discussed further in Chapter 2 on essential stretching also lead to some persistently weak areas that need some attention with focused core work. While the quadriceps (at the front of the thigh) can often become dominant, the gluteals (buttock muscles) and upper hamstrings can become relatively weak. Although the glutes can significantly contribute to power output and ground speed when you work harder, particular when climbing or sprinting at speed, for most of the time they do not make a significant contribution to the cycling movement relative to the muscles at the front of the thighs. This will be particularly true for a cyclist who has not been athletic or 'sporty' prior to taking up cycling, as the glutes are most developed with multidirectional running games, sprinting or strength training.

'Quadriceps dominance' is a term used to describe when the quads at the front of the thigh become overdeveloped and overactive relative to the posterior muscles, namely the gluteals (or buttocks) and often the upper hamstrings. Characteristically, the quads will be strong and will try to do all the work, while the gluteals which are often weaker, will need some encouragement to become active. Cyclists with this pattern of muscle recruitment will often be more likely to experience cramp in the thighs, and in particular suffer problems in the ITB, or knee pain because of the subsequent mal-tracking of the knee cap that can result. In practice, the best way to tackle the problem is to combine pre-stretching of the tight areas of the quads (as explained in Chapter 2) followed immediately by strengthening of the gluteals and upper hamstrings, using some of hip extension exercises described here.

The relatively low-level recruitment of the glute muscles in cyclists is a perfectly natural way for the body to adapt to lower to moderate intensity cycling. In a sense it's testament to your body's efficiency that it will only use the muscles it needs to produce the speed or power necessary at any given time. As powerful explosive muscles, the glutes are generally not suited to working for really long periods at moderate intensities as is characteristic of most cycling. Furthermore, in the cycling movement they are working in a lengthened range and never fully shorten as they would in sprint running, for example, where the leg

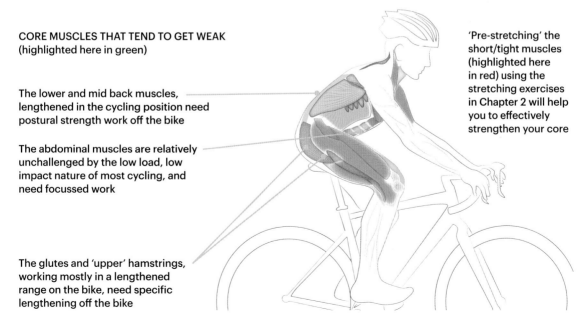

CORE MUSCLES THAT TEND TO GET WEAK
(highlighted here in green)

The lower and mid back muscles, lengthened in the cycling position need postural strength work off the bike

The abdominal muscles are relatively unchallenged by the low load, low impact nature of most cycling, and need focussed work

The glutes and 'upper' hamstrings, working mostly in a lengthened range on the bike, need specific lengthening off the bike

'Pre-stretching' the short/tight muscles (highlighted here in red) using the stretching exercises in Chapter 2 will help you to effectively strengthen your core

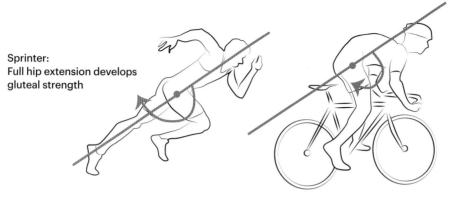

Sprinter:
Full hip extension develops gluteal strength

Cyclist:
Partial hip extension means gluteal strength must be developed off the bike

drives behind the line of the torso for maximum hip extension as the sprinter gets out of the blocks and into full stride. Instead, both in and out of the saddle on the bike, the range of movement for the glutes is limited. This is one of the strongest arguments for including off-the-bike conditioning work for you to develop the glute strength you need for those times on the bike when you really need these most powerful hip muscles.

My essential core exercises for the hips and back focus on the areas that tend to weaken at low and moderate intensities on the bike, or that work in a lengthened range at various stages in the cycling pedal stroke. In particular, some of the exercises here will target the glutes and upper hamstrings. Isolating these muscle areas off the bike maintains the strength and tone needed for optimal performance at higher intensities on the bike, when these muscle groups are more likely to be recruited.

It's fairly broadly understood that weak glute muscles can contribute to lack of strength on the bike and also pain and problems, particularly in the knees. In my view, because of the biomechanical disadvantage that the glute muscles have when on the bike, this strengthening has to be done off the bike, but can be supported by cycling-specific elements that help to integrate your new-found strength as your core muscle balance improves. With all the will in the world, just thinking about engaging your glutes as you ride your bike will not do it.

To maximize the benefit of the core exercises in this chapter, integrating the bike drills that help to stimulate and refine the timing and recruitment of your core muscles through the cycling action at higher intensities is recommended. A detailed discussion of what these might be is outside the scope of this book, but will get a mention later in Chapter 6 on periodization and planning.

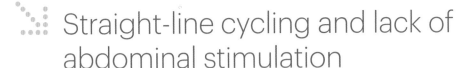

Straight-line cycling and lack of abdominal stimulation

In addition to the weakening of certain muscles along the back of the body, the abdominal muscles of a cyclist's core are relatively unchallenged by most cycling. More typically stimulated and tested by ground forces with walking and running, and with multidimensional strength movements such as lunging, pushing, pulling and twisting, a cyclist's abdominals can become relatively inactive. Only coming into play more significantly at higher intensities, or when you stand out of the saddle to more actively push and pull on the bars, relative to other sports and to our primal template, the cycling position can lead to weakness in the abdominal muscles. When cycling, it's possible to rest your body on the bars and drive hard with the legs with very little involvement of the abdominal muscles, save for their movement in allowing for deep breathing. Again, this can lead to problems at the point at which you want to ramp up the intensity of your riding or add more explosive elements that need your abs to be alert and working in the way they should.

Lack of abdominal strength may lead to changes in your pedalling style at higher intensities, such as your knees rolling inwards towards the top tube or your hips and lower back rocking and rolling in the saddle. You may experience pain or discomfort in your back or knees with hard, out of the saddle efforts, or you may just feel unable to produce the power you want on the flat during hard efforts, disproportionate to how efficient you feel at a constant and steadier cycling speed.

Balance, as a separate skill to 'core balance', should be distinguished here. Some people believe that someone with good balance must have a great core but this is not technically correct. Balance is for the most part a proprioceptive movement skill that can be developed independent of an optimally functioning core. When I talk about 'core balance' here, I am referring to the muscles around the core being well balanced in their tension, length and ability to contract at the right time and in the right way with any given movement. It's true that having well-balanced core muscles may help you learn to balance on the bike as a cycling skill, but it's not a given. Equally, some cyclists who have exceptional balance skills on their bike may not have well-balanced core muscles.

'Inner' and 'outer' abdominals

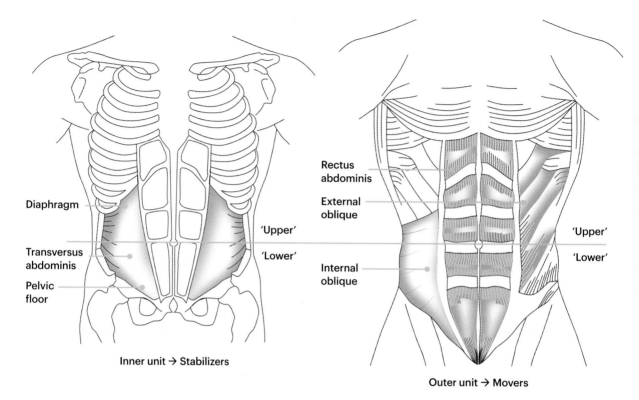

Diaphragm

Transversus
abdominis

Pelvic
floor

'Upper'

'Lower'

Inner unit → Stabilizers

Rectus
abdominis

External
oblique

Internal
oblique

'Upper'

'Lower'

Outer unit → Movers

The functional anatomy of the abdominal muscles and how they relate and connect with the other muscles that cross the core is quite complex, allowing for both stability and movement in three dimensions. The deepest abdominal muscle, the transversus abdominus, or 'TVA' as it is sometimes called, has had some publicity – because of its stabilizing function, a weak TVA is often blamed for back injuries. This belt-like muscle engages as you draw your navel in, and works together with the muscles of the pelvic floor and diaphragm (which sits under your ribs), as an 'inner unit' team of stabilizers. Layered on top of these muscles are the internal and external obliques, and the rectus abdominus muscle (the most superficial 'six-pack' muscle), which have a role in moving and generating force through your core. These more superficial muscles might be called an 'outer unit', as they predominantly work as movers rather than stabilizers, although there are exceptions to that general rule.

In referring to 'inner' or 'outer' abdominal muscles here I am using the terms to help you understand broadly their complex role in both stability and movement.

For some people, getting a sense of how to engage the inner unit of muscles can be difficult. Often, if these muscles have become weak or relatively 'shut off' for some time, re-establishing a neuromuscular connection with them can be difficult. You might find you are concentrating hard on engaging them the way you are told, but can't actually *feel* anything happening. Pilates-style exercises and those prescribed by physiotherapists are often targeting the deeper 'inner' abdominals and may make you feel like you are not actually *doing* anything. I have not overemphasized highly technical 'inner unit' exercises here, as they are often difficult to grasp without one-to-one coaching from someone trained in clinical exercise, like a physiotherapist or a specialist Pilates instructor.

The abdominal exercises in this chapter are focused on getting the abdominal group of muscles to work well as a whole, working both the 'inner' and 'outer' muscles. If you struggle with your alignment or position with these exercises, or can't tell what you are supposed to be doing to get your abdominal muscles to engage, I recommend you seek one-to-one help from a physiotherapist, a corrective exercise specialist like myself, or a Pilates instructor trained in clinical or rehab-type exercise.

As is the case with activating the glute muscles, I believe that focused abdominal exercises are essential off the bike to restore some of the normal multidimensional stability that you don't get on the bike or seated at your desk. You should not have to think about engaging your core when you ride, it should just happen naturally, but ensuring that your muscles are working as they should may take some time and effort. There have been some ideas in cycling circles that 'thinking about' engaging your glutes or your abdominals when cycling will help you to develop a stronger core, but in my experience this is not the case. If you want to develop a functional core on the bike, you have to work it off the bike first, and then integrate that strength and control on the bike later.

The essential abdominal exercises included here challenge all three planes of movement to ensure that you develop multidimensional abdominal strength. They include more static stabilizing exercises to stimulate the 'inner' abdominals, and some more dynamic moving exercises to strengthen the 'outer' abdominals. Conditioning both ensures that your abdominals can support you in their postural endurance role (when riding for long periods, for example) as well as in their dynamic strength role (at higher intensities on the bike as well as in functional lifting movements off the bike).

Using Swiss balls for big bang benefits

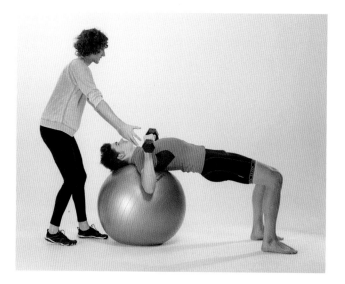

In this chapter the Swiss ball really comes into its own to help to stimulate your core to become active because of its inherent instability. Compared to similar core exercises performed on the floor, or another stable surface, I have found that Swiss ball exercises are more likely to encourage good form by way of 'waking up' core muscles that may otherwise have been dormant for some time. Where your body has got used to cycling (which most of the time has low core demands), it may need a 'kick' to wake up those muscles that you are trying to engage to bring about better muscle balance. In particular, if you tend to be hypermobile, the Swiss ball options in this chapter will be the better choices for you to ensure that multiple muscles become active and that you are not overstressing one joint.

A 'big bang' exercise is a term I have borrowed from Paul Chek and refers to exercises that give you many benefits in one go. Several of the Swiss ball exercise in this chapter give you a big bang of benefits, working multiple muscles in one exercise in many dimensions, as well as stimulating your balance and control. You will know a big bang exercise when you encounter one because it will make you quite hot quite quickly!

Standing posture as core training in itself

Towards the end of this chapter I include an example of a light bicep curl for postural training and standing awareness. I've included this example as an important precursor to the more loaded strength exercises in Chapter 3, where maintaining good upright alignment is essential to practising an exercise with good form. Many cyclists have poor posture because they are not used to moving in an upright way as part of their sport or fitness. Sometimes poor posture is simply a matter of body awareness, and can be easily remedied by relearning how to stand upright. In other instances, poor posture is a combination of lack of awareness and muscle imbalance syndromes or stiffness in the spine acting on the body to pull it into a particular position.

Some of the common muscle imbalances seen in cyclists have been discussed already, but their impact on your standing posture becomes particularly important when you start to load your body in an upright position. Before adding any weight to any of the strength exercises in Chapter 3 in particular, it's important to be able to adopt an upright posture with a neutral spine, where the curves of the spine are well balanced so that the whole body is taking the load of the exercise to achieve the desired result.

Straight vs neutral: Although you may have heard the word 'straight' as a technique cue when exercising, the spine should never actually be straight. To 'stand up straight' actually means having the spine in its natural, 'neutral' position. The postural curves are dynamic and can change with movement, but an upright spine is more correctly described as 'neutral' because the natural anatomical curves help the body function when loaded from this position.

I have included these 'standing posture trainers' at the end of this essential core chapter to prepare you for the more upright loading that your body will experience in the essential strength exercises is Chapter 3. These standing exercises can help you relearn good posture and represent a transitional exercise towards including more strength work in your programme. I will explain in more detail how to include appropriate exercises from each chapter in Chapter 6, on periodization and programme design.

Here I am using a dowel rod as an indicator of alignment in the standing biceps curl. Later I will show you how to use a doorframe to give you some feedback as to how you are standing, and whether you are ready to add load in the strength exercises in Chapter 3.

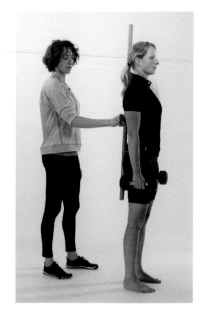

Good posture and axial loading

I have introduced the idea of a neutral spine in Chapter 3 already in relation to the importance of good alignment in the essential strength exercises there. For some cyclists it may take some time before good upright alignment is possible, and the key to changing your posture and being able to establish and maintain a neutral spine during loaded movement is having a strong and balanced core. Throughout this chapter you will see repeated emphasis on correct alignment, particularly in the abdominal exercises where I emphasize the importance of a neutral spine the most.

Axial loading is the application of weight or force along the long axis of the body. In conditioning terms, it refers to any upright exercise where you are adding significant load by carrying weight, which places compressive emphasis on the spine, hips and pelvis. In these type of exercises: lunges, squats and dead lifts, the core must be stable so that the muscles and joints are sharing the load effectively to generate force without causing injury.

You will see me using a dowel rod or stick along the spine in the horse stance exercises to give you an idea of what 'neutral' should look like, and in the standing posture trainer at the end I explain how you can use an open doorframe to get a sense of your standing postural alignment too. Having good alignment as described throughout these exercises is an important precursor to adding any significant load in the strength essentials in Chapter 3. If you find that you are struggling to adopt the posture described here, don't worry. Get as close as you can at the stage that you are at and keep working away at the flexibility and core essentials in particular to continue progressing.

For some cyclists, good posture or a neutral alignment may take some time to achieve due to long-established muscle imbalances and restrictions that need to be unravelled. Don't be disheartened if you find some of these positions difficult to achieve. Simply continue working on the essential conditioning elements in this book in a varied and periodized way, and you will find that with persistence your body will start to change.

Assessing your posture with a view to working with weights

The more you struggle to achieve good posture and alignment with the core essentials in this chapter, the more you need to be aware of your alignment when choosing to include some of the strength essentials from Chapter 3. However, that does not mean that you should not include them, just that you should choose the option that you can do well and keep coming back to those that are more difficult to see how you have improved after a period of training. The key to long-term changes in your condition and performance is maintaining a consistent, balanced and varied approach to your training, which allows you to improve month on month, year on year.

Chapter 6 on periodization and planning will help you understand how to select exercises that are most appropriate to you at any given time, and help you progress and improve your performance month on month and year on year. (By working with those exercises that you can do well, and coming back to those that you initially find too difficult, you will eventually be able to perform more of the exercises in this book effectively to develop a well-rounded and varied conditioning programme.)

Repetitions, sets and rest periods

The repetitions, sets and rest periods in this chapter are quite different to those in Chapter 3 on essential strength training. Many of the exercises here are designed to increase core stability, and for some of the muscles of the back and abdominals in particular, that will be best achieved by holding certain positions, or moving slowly. Depending on what type of strength you are trying to achieve in a particular movement or muscle group, you can manipulate these variables for different desired results.

A detailed discussion of the science of intensity, repetitions, sets and rest periods is outside the scope of this book. In this chapter on essential core exercises, I have focused on how the exercises should be performed and taken a simple approach to these other variables. Some of the exercises include isometric holds (see below) to maximize the development of postural endurance, an aspect of core fitness particularly important to cyclists. The rest periods are often deliberately shorter too, to maximize postural and core muscle endurance.

An 'isometric' exercise is one where the length of the muscle does not change throughout the movement. Most movements have a concentric phase (when the muscle is shortening under load) and an eccentric phase (when the muscle is lengthening against a load). An isometric exercise is one where the position is deliberately held at some point in this movement. In this chapter, two examples of isometric exercises are the prone cobra for strengthening the lower and mid-back muscles, and the Swiss ball side lead for strengthening the abdominal muscles along the sides of the body.

Some of the isometric exercises in this chapter develop maximal 'time under tension' in the weakest part of the muscles, where we are trying to have the biggest impact. Consequently, they might feel quite different to exercises that you are used to, and can be particularly tough. There will be progressions towards longer holds rather than adding heavier load, or more resistance, with the primary goal being better endurance rather than greater pure strength. Focusing on getting in the best possible position you can and progressively working through the stages will give you the best results, rather than rushing straight to the longer holds.

Some of the exercises have both an isometric variation (such as with the Swiss ball side lean) and a more dynamic version (as with the Swiss ball side bend), encouraging you to develop stability first, then strength in the movement second. It's worth working through the exercises in sequence here to ensure you achieve the best form. As part of your periodization you should then cycle through the exercise options to ensure you get a good balance of core stability and core strength.

The Essential Core Exercises

 ## Strengthening the back of the body

I have broadly separated the exercises in this chapter into exercises for the back and front of the body. The exercises for the front of the body can be split further into those that strengthen the postural muscles of the lower and upper back, and those that strengthen the cycling muscles more, i.e. the glutes and upper hamstrings. You will see that the exercises targeting the cycling muscles will tend to have an 8–12 repetitions range, while the exercises targeting the postural muscles will have progressive isometric holds. In some exercises there will be some crossover between the two.

Hip and lower back extensions (glutes, upper hamstrings and lower back)

The first of my essential core exercises targets the glutes (buttocks), upper hamstrings and lower back, although all the muscles along the back of the body are involved in the movement. Hip extension exercises are great for strengthening the glutes and back, taking the body into the fully extended position that it never achieves when cycling or sitting. I have chosen this Swiss ball supine hip extension because there is room for progression towards tougher exercises as you get stronger, with no other equipment. Also, the instability of the ball helps to 'wake up' sleepy glutes and engage the back and abdominal muscles of the trunk. The more advanced 'hip extension with knee bend' version of the exercise has some cycling-specific carry-over too, as it is 'open chain' with the legs moving away from and back towards the hips, just as they do when you ride your bike. Targeting these areas in a focused and isolated way can ensure the development of strength in these areas and help you engage these powerful muscles on the bike.

From a cycling standpoint, weakness in the glutes is probably the single-most limiting factor in terms of muscle strength connected to power output, particularly when you start to work harder and push towards and above your threshold. As prime movers at the hips on the downstroke, the glutes come into play particularly with sprints and accelerations, or for time-trial type efforts along the flat where the pelvis naturally tips forwards. For many cyclists the glutes need activating, so this hip extension is essential in reminding them how to work and get stronger.

To achieve the biggest benefit from these exercises you should pre-stretch/mobilize the areas that tend to be tight/stiff along the back of the body. These may include the piriformis, lower hamstrings and thoracic spine. Check these exercises from Chapter 2 on essential stretching to see whether you need to perform these stretches to maximize the benefits.

Swiss ball hip extension feet on ball

Arms out to sides

Preparation

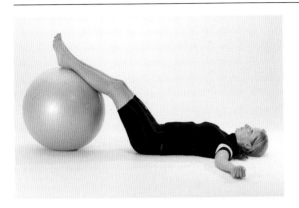

Lie with your legs on the ball and your arms outstretched at your sides, level with your shoulders. To start with, keep the ball close to your hips so that both your calves and the back of your hamstrings are touching the ball.

Movement

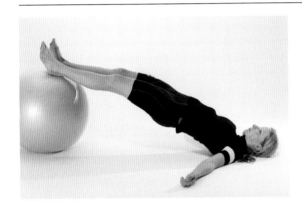

Push down with your legs and lift your hips and chest *as high as you can*, drawing your navel in as you move, and squeezing your glutes at the top of the movement. Hold the top position (aiming for your shoulder, hip, knee and ankle to be in one straight line) for 5 seconds before returning your hips to the floor with control. It is very important that you achieve this straight line position to properly engage your glutes before progressing the exercise further.

If you find you are able to perform the maximum number of repetitions and sets with good form, with the ball quite close to your body, start with it a little further away from you. Small changes in the distance between your hips and the top of the ball can make a significant difference in the difficulty of this exercise, so progress gradually until your heels are on the top of the ball (as shown here). Alternatively, you can progress this exercise by choosing the more unstable option on the next page, with your arms across your chest.

Arms across chest

Preparation

Lie with your legs on the ball as before, but with your arms across your chest. To start with, keep the ball close to your hips so that both your calves and the back of your hamstrings are touching the ball.

Movement

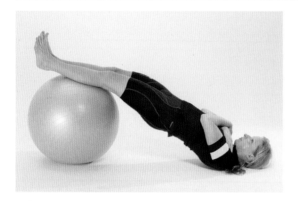

Push down with your legs and lift your hips and chest as high as you can, drawing your navel in as you move, and squeezing your glutes at the top of the movement. Hold the top position (aiming for your shoulder, hip, knee and ankle to be in a straight line) for 5 seconds before returning your hips to the floor with control. It is very important that you achieve this straight line position to properly engage your glutes before progressing the exercise further. This variation of the exercise is much more unstable, since your base of support is significantly reduced by taking your arms across your chest. This makes it a good variation if you are keen to emphasize the stability benefits of the exercise in addition to simply strengthening the glutes and back of the body.

If you find you are able to perform the maximum number of repetitions and sets with good form, with the ball quite close to your body, start with it a little further away from you. Small changes in the distance between your hips and the top of the ball can make a significant difference in the difficulty of this exercise, so progress gradually until your heels are on the top of the ball (opposite). Once you are able to achieve this variation with good form for the maximum number of reps and sets, you can progress by trying the hip extension with knee bend variation opposite.

Hip extension with knee bend sequence

This advanced variation of this exercise should only be attempted once you have mastered the previous two variations and worked on them consistently for 8–12 weeks. The increase in challenge with the hip extension with knee bend is quite a jump in difficulty, so I recommend you perform as many repetitions of this exercise as you can do well, and then finish your set with the previous variation.

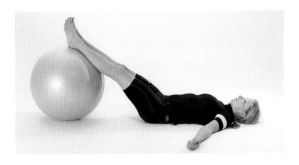

Preparation

Lie with your legs on the ball and your arms outstretched at your sides, level with your shoulders. To allow room for the knee bend you need your heels to be on the top of the ball, as shown.

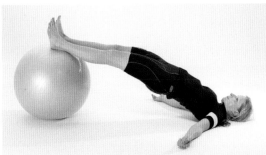

Movement

Push down with your legs and lift your hips and chest *as high as you can*, drawing your navel in as you move and squeezing your glutes at the top of the movement. This top position – with your shoulder, hip, knee and ankle in one straight line – then becomes the start and finish position for each of the knee bend repetitions. From here, dig your heels hard into the ball and lift your hips further as you bend your knees and pull the ball towards you. Your hips must lift up higher as you do this, so that throughout the movement, your shoulders, hips and knees stay in a straight line.

From this high position (shown centre left) slowly extend back out to the start position, ensuring that your hips don't dip as you do so. Repeat this movement as many times as you can, finishing the set with one of the previous variations if you need to.

How many reps and sets?

Perform 8–12 repetitions for 2–3 sets, with 30 seconds' rest between sets. Choose the variation that you can do with good form and work on it for 8–12 weeks before progressing to a new level of the exercise.

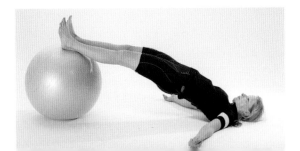

Upper and lower back extensions (lower back, upper back and shoulders)

The exercises in this chapter for the upper and lower back are essential since they tackle a cyclist's postural tendencies towards hunched and rounded shoulders and a flattened lumbar curve or lower back. This poor posture can make you susceptible to injuries that can force you off the bike, as well as limiting power potential by changing the position of your hips and back on the bike.

Both the exercises in this section are truly 'corrective' in that they both strengthen the weak areas of the back and hips and at the same time help to mobilize the tight areas that can be restrictive. When performed together with the thoracic foam roller exercise in particular, these exercises can have a profound effect on your back strength, posture and cycling performance.

The prone cobra

The prone cobra works all the muscles along the back of the body, but notably isolates the upper-back muscles. The way the exercise is performed here, with the thumbs turned backwards, also works the external rotator cuff muscles of the shoulder, which can become weak through hours spent holding the bars. As you sit reading this, visualize the position of your upper back and arms as you hold the 'tops' of the handlebars, and then reverse that position, lifting your chest, extending your back and turning your thumbs backwards. It should literally be the exact opposite position.

Because this is a 'postural exercise', it is best performed with progressively prolonged isometric holds. As you develop more endurance in these muscles you can increase the duration of the held position and reduce the rest in between each repetition. The ultimate goal is three minutes' time under tension in total, broken down into progressively longer holds with fewer 'sets' to perform.

The prone cobra restores basic levels of postural strength to your back. Your bike fit can improve with regular use of this exercise too, as it will allow you to achieve a 'flatter' or more stretched out aerodynamic position. Lower back injuries and shoulder impingement problems can also be kept at bay with the prone cobra.

Off the floor

Preparation

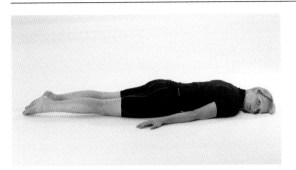

Start by lying flat on your front, head turned to one side, and your arms at the sides of your body, with your little fingers close to your sides and thumbs pointing away from you.

Movement

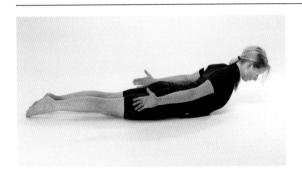

Lift your upper back off the floor, turning your thumbs backwards as you move, and squeezing your shoulder blades together. The goal is to turn the arms backwards as much as possible, keeping them close to your sides and stretching the front of your chest. Leave your legs on the floor if you can, and keep your neck long at the back so that your chin is tucked in and you look down towards the floor. Focus in extending the most through your upper back, by arching through the upper back and opening your chest forwards.

Swiss ball variation

This Swiss ball variation of the same exercise feels slightly different but fundamentally works on the same areas. Because of their role in stabilizing the ball, the hip and glute muscles become more active in this variation too, which may make it a better option for some. Overall, this prone cobra offers a *bigger bang*, working the mid and upper back, but also the lower back, glutes and hamstrings.

Preparation

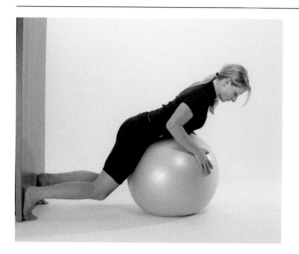

Position the ball underneath your hips (as shown), with your feet resting against a wall where it meets the floor. Your feet should be a little wider than hip width to give you a solid base from which to move.

Movement

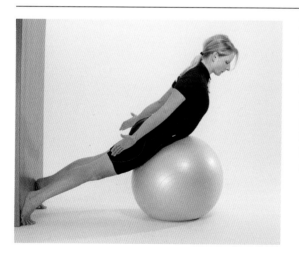

Press your hips into the ball, engaging your glutes and tucking your hips down, raising your body into the prone cobra position by extending your back and turning your arms backwards. Your arms should stay close to your body, but you should rotate them backwards from the shoulder as much as you can. In this variation of the exercise it's important that you extend evenly and don't 'hinge' at any point in the lower back. If you feel this exercise is uncomfortable in the lower back, you may not be engaging your glutes enough, so focus on pressing your hips into the ball strongly to avoid this.

Wide arms variation

This Swiss ball wide arm variation of the prone cobra uses the weight of the outstretched arm to increase the challenge to the mid-back muscles, to match the added load to the hips but choosing to work on the ball. It is the hardest of the variations here, and can be made even more challenging by carrying a light dumbbell in each hand. A weight of only 1kg can make this a really challenging exercise for the muscles of the mid-back and the external rotator cuff.

Preparation

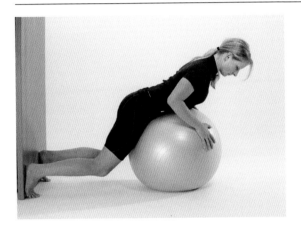

Position the ball underneath your hips (as shown), with your feet resting against a wall where it meets the floor. Your feet should be a little wider than hip width to give you a solid base from which to move.

Movement

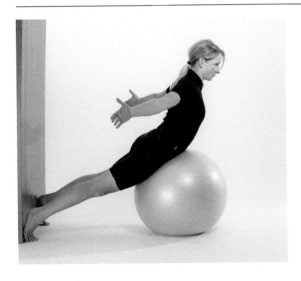

Press your hips into the ball, engaging your glutes and tucking your hips down, raising your body into the prone cobra position by extending your back and turning your arms backwards. Take your arms wide, so that they are level with, or slightly below, your shoulders, rotating your arms backwards from the shoulder as much as you can by turning the thumb backwards and upwards. In this variation of the exercise it's important that your arms are at least level with your body, if not slightly behind the line of your body (as shown), to emphasize the work to the mid-back muscles. If you feel this exercise is uncomfortable in the lower back, you may not be engaging your glutes enough, so focus on pressing your hips into the ball strongly to avoid this.

How many reps and sets?

Since this is a 'postural exercise' the progressions focus on longer holds for the isometric position, with progressively shorter rest periods. In the set descriptions below, 'on' means that you are in the position, and 'off' means that you come out of the position.

Suggested progressions to work through are:

3 × 20 seconds on 10 seconds off × 2–3 sets

3 × 30 seconds on 15 seconds off × 2 sets

3 × 45 seconds on, 15 seconds off × 2 sets

3 × 1 minute held with 30 seconds' rest × 1 set

Though it may be tempting to go straight to the 'harder' sets here, it is more sensible to work through the progressions and focus on the quality of the position (staying as high as you can, turning your thumbs right back, and squeezing your shoulder blades together).

Working through the floor-based prone cobra for 8–12 weeks before progressing to a new level of the exercise is usually a good idea. The only exception is for riders who tend to be hypermobile, where the Swiss ball versions may feel more comfortable straight away.

Extension with rotation

This next sequence of exercise variations strengthens the muscles of the back while restoring movement in rotation. The variations also help restore some cross-patterning movements that keep a human nervous system wired for movement. When performed together with the thoracic foam roller exercise in particular, these exercises can have a profound effect on your back strength and mobility. If you found that in working through the essential stretching exercises your upper back mobility was particularly poor, including one of these exercises will help you re-establish mobility and core strength together.

'Cross-patterning' or 'cross-crawling' movements remind the nervous system how to coordinate the left and right sides of the body. As humans, we are designed to move 'contralaterally'. That is to say as the right leg swings back (as we walk for example) the left arm swings back, and vice versa. On a bike, this natural cross-patterning does not happen. In fact, if anything we function with an ipsilateral (same side) movement: as the left leg pushes down (and back) the left arm pulls on the bars. For cyclists who often consider themselves uncoordinated off the bike, reminding the body of this all-important contralateral coordination can help you move better in general, and can open up cross-training options too.

Alternating superman

The alternating superman exercise works diagonally across the core to coordinate and balance strength in the left hip and right back and vice versa respectively. It can help to highlight asymmetries in the 'posterior sling' of muscles from one hip to the opposing side of your upper body. Many human movements require correct coordination and timing of the left and right sides of the body, not least in the arm swing when we walk or run, but also when we push and pull objects as we stand on our feet.

The alternating superman helps cyclists maintain the left-right coordination that is important in many sports and activities, but is largely absent from cycling. It also helps restore mobility in the upper back at the same time as improving strength.

Off the floor

Preparation

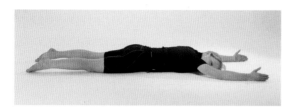

Start by lying flat on your front with your head turned to one side and your arms outstretched overhead. Your thumbs should be turned up for this exercise (as shown).

Movement

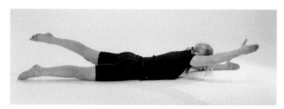

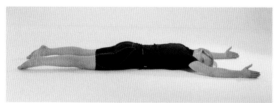

Moving from the shoulder and hip with a straight arm and leg, raise your right arm and your left leg off the floor, trying to match the height of your arm to the height of your leg, and lifting your upper body with your arm just enough to allow for the movement. Keep your chin tucked in and your eyes looking down, so that the back of your neck is in line with your upper back. At the same time as you are lifting your arm and leg, stretch one away from the other so that you feel you are stretching your spine and making the line from your toes to your fingertips as long as possible.

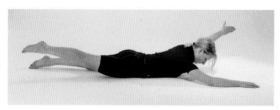

Hold the best possible position you can with determination for 5 seconds, before lowering and then repeating on the opposite diagonal. Move into position slowly and steadily and focus on the quality of the movement using the technique points here.

Swiss ball variation

The Swiss ball variation of this exercise represents a considerable balance challenge as compared to the floor exercise. It may take some practice before you find you are able to do this exercise at all, but if you keep working at it you will find you can eventually come into an effective alternating superman position.

Preparation

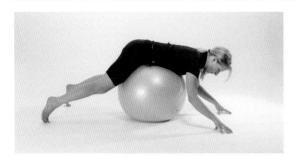

Lie flat over your ball and spread your hands and feet into a rectangular square shape, using your cupped fingers and your toes to get a sense of how your weight is distributed across all four points. Try to balance such that your weight is evenly distributed across all four before you start to move.

Movement

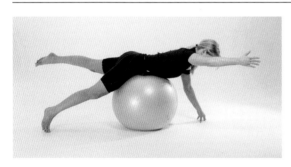

Moving slowly so that you can respond reflexively to the change in balance on the ball, start to raise your right arm and your left leg. Counterbalance one with the other as you move towards a position where your opposite arm and leg are extended in line with your body. You will notice that if you raise your leg too quickly in particular, you will roll forwards on the ball. This is because your leg is much heavier than your arm. It pays to raise your leg steadily and slowly, so that it doesn't get ahead of your arm. Once extended, hold the lengthened position for 5 seconds as best you can, before lowering your right arm and left leg and swapping sides, as shown middle and bottom.

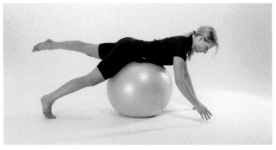

How many reps and sets?

Perform 8–12 repetitions for 2–3 sets, with 30 seconds' rest between sets. Choose one of these exercises and work on it for 8–12 weeks, before changing to the other variation.

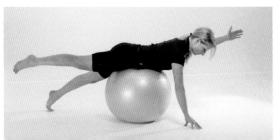

Strengthening the front and sides of the body

The next selection of exercises predominantly strengthens the front of the body, notably the abdominal muscles. However, no exercise here only works one muscle at a time, or exclusively one dimension, and so muscles of the hips and back will get involved too, linking the front of the body with the other muscles surrounding the core.

Core without flexion

'Core without flexion' is a concept I use as a catchphrase to allow cyclists, and others, to grasp the idea and practicality of strengthening the abdominal muscles without overemphasizing flexion. A flexion movement is any movement where you bend forwards, and many abdominal exercises, like traditional crunches off the floor, rely on this movement to contract the abdominals into their shortened range. While there will always be exceptions to the rule, overemphasis on exercises like the traditional sit-up can lead to problems for cyclists, since they are already stiff along the back of the body, and the muscles of the upper abdomen in particular can be short due to poor posture through the upper back and prolonged periods spent bent over the bike. An additional concern is that many cyclists have a flattened lower back or lumbar spine, and some may be at risk of lumbar disc injuries with excessive flexion exercises. Although this may only refer to a minority, if there are safer and more effective alternatives it makes sense to use them to avoid this sometimes serious injury.

Wanting to avoid flexion presents a problem for cyclists who want to strengthen their abdominals without worsening their posture by excessively shortening the 'upper' abdominals in particular. My proposed solution to this problem is to avoid flexion as much as possible, and instead work in all other dimensions while maintaining a 'neutral spine', or by bending or twisting in the frontal (sideways) and transverse (twisting) planes.

The only exceptions in this chapter are the Swiss ball crunch and the lower body Russian twist with cross crunch. The Swiss ball crunch includes lumbar flexion, but with full hyperextension by way of a backwards bend over the ball between each repetition, while the lower body twist with cross crunch includes a full rotational stretch between repetitions. These exceptions have an inherent flexibility element to help maintain flexibility while developing strength, but should still be avoided if you know you have a history of lumbar disc problems.

'Flexion dominance' is a term used to describe the tendency of many people (cyclists included) to have many more forwards bending movements in their day-to-day lives than backwards bending ones. Excessive 'flexion' movements in your daily or weekly movement vocabulary can cause problems, so training the core without excessive flexion becomes an important goal if you are looking to restore balance and optimal performance.

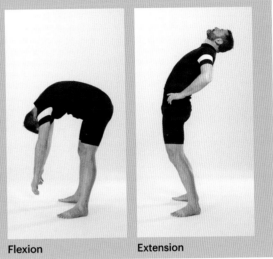

Flexion   **Extension**

Four-point exercises for stability and 'inner units'

The variations on four-point exercises in this next section are designed to strengthen the 'inner unit' of the abdominals (the transversus abdominis and pelvic floor muscles), but also the 'inner units' of the hip and shoulder joints. Both the hips and shoulders are very mobile and depend on a 'rotator cuff' of deeper stabilizing muscles to hold the joints in place, while the larger muscles crossing the joint generate force and movement.

Joints need to be 'stable' in order for force to be transmitted across them, and so working on the intrinsic 'stability' of the spine, hips and shoulders is important if you want to maximize your potential for force generation on the bike. Where stability is poor, your body will limit the amount of power that crosses the joints in order to avoid injury, and so without adequate stability your performance gains will be limited.

Some of the best exercises for focused stability work on your shoulders, hips and trunk are what I call 'horse stance' exercises, or 'table top' variations. I learned the importance of these horse-stance exercises through my training with the CHEK institute, but they also form a staple of traditional and clinical Pilates exercises. These exercises performed on all fours provide a 'big bang' of stability benefits to all these important areas in one hit.

They are often considered 'rehab' or 'prehab' exercises, and refer back to the fundamental core fitness we develop in the trunk, shoulders and hips through crawling as babies and young children. Working through the core with the opposing arm and leg action develops the stability we need for more powerful movements later on, and can also maintain your shoulder and hip stability in the minimum time.

Since the glutes are key drivers of the legs, stability at the sides of your hips in particular can help you maintain 'neutral' alignment with your legs as you pedal, rather than having your knee roll in and out with the up and down action. Weakness in the gluteus medius muscle (the lateral glute on the side of your hip) is often implicated in knee problems and these four-point exercises teach you how to activate this area before subsequently integrating that strength into movements such as those in Chapter 3 of this book.

Equally, shoulder stability is important on the bike too. As you hold the bars for hours on end you are stabilizing against the force generated by the legs to ensure no effort is wasted and to avoid inefficient and unnecessary shoulder movements. When you stand out of the saddle, stability in the shoulder gives you the potential to generate force efficiently through your arms and core, adding to the more direct power you generate through your legs and hips.

It may seem like a bit of a leap to understand how floor exercises performed on all fours can benefit your riding, but stability of the hips and shoulders (as well as the abdomen) is really important. Training the lateral stabilizers of the hips to maintain knee stability and the rotator cuff of the shoulder to maintain shoulder stability, these exercises should be a priority if you have any knee or shoulder problems that get in the way of your riding.

Horse stances

This type of exercise can be difficult to get a grip of if you prefer doing everything at speed, or don't see the training benefit unless something 'hurts'. It's important to take your time to understand what you are trying to do and how your body should feel if you want to really see the benefits. This first variation – the horse stance vertical – provides the foundation for all the subsequent variations, so don't skip it before progressing to the others, particularly if you haven't tried this type of exercise before.

Vertical

Every other variation of the horse stance described here should start with this fundamental 'hover' position, which provides the foundation for all other movements of the arms and legs. This variation of the exercise challenges the transverse plane (twisting) the most.

Preparation

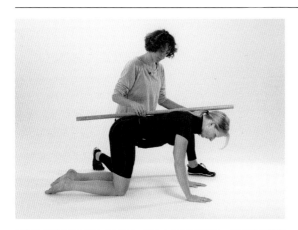

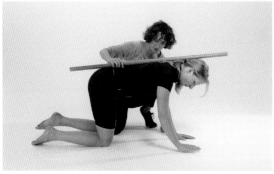

Start with your knees under your hips and your hands under your shoulders so that you are making a rectangular shape with all four points on the floor underneath you. Then soften your elbows, tucking them in, and make sure that your back is neither rounded like a cat or excessively dipped in the back like a cow. Ideally you should have a shallow dip in your lower back, but otherwise your hip, shoulder and ear should be all in one line.

To practise correct alignment, you can use a dowel rod or pole balanced along your spine to check for three points of contact – at the pelvis, between the shoulder blades and the back of your head. Your gaze should fall between your hands with your chin tucked in so that your neck is in line with the rest of your body. If you slide your hand between the pole and your lower back (as shown overleaf), you can adjust your position so that you have just enough space to slide the thickness of your hand into the gap, and also the correct contact points along your back. Although this technique takes some patience, it can make a massive difference to how effectively you are able to perform this exercise.

When I work one to one with clients, I use a dowel rod along the spine to check for neutral alignment and to provide feedback.

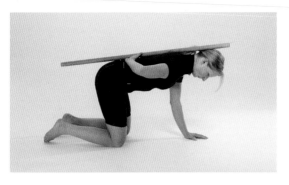 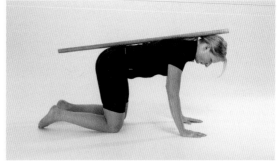

Minimal movement

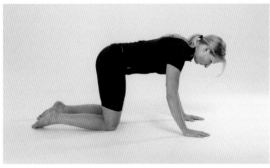

Once in position, take a full breath into your tummy and as you breathe out, draw your navel in towards your spine to maintain engagement of the deep core muscles. It should feel like you have pulled in a thick corset-like belt around your lower belly. Progressively press one hand and the opposite knee into the ground until you find you are hovering on the opposite diagonal.

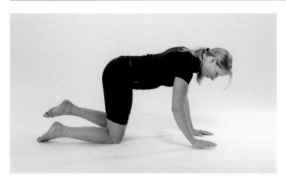

Hold this hover position for 5 seconds, before lowering and changing sides. Your goal is to keep your body as still as possible throughout, keeping your core engaged by drawing your belly button in and holding your supporting shoulder and hip steady. You should be able to feel your middle working hard to hold you steady, and may find as the repetitions go on that you start to 'shake' a little to hold position, which indicates that your muscles are working and beginning to fatigue.

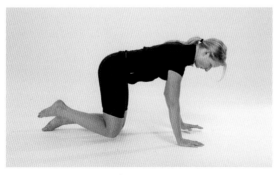

Horizontal

The horse stance horizontal takes the opposite arm and leg into an outstretched position similar to that of the alternating superman exercise described earlier. This variation of the exercise challenges the sagittal plane (forwards and backwards bending) the most.

Movement

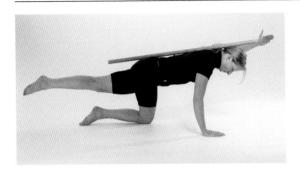

Drawing your navel in to stabilize, and pushing down on the supporting hand and knee, slowly extend your opposite arm and leg, taking them along the line of your body (level with your hip with your leg, and slightly outside your shoulder for your arm) until they are outstretched and in line with your body. Your goal with this exercise is to move as far as you can without any change in the shape of your core. If your back dips in at the lower back or you round your upper back you have lost your alignment or gone too far into the position. Once you have gone as far as you can and maintained your core alignment, hold the position for 5 seconds before lowering your arm and leg and changing sides.

Abduction

The horse stance abduction takes the leg and arm to the sides of the body, challenging the frontal (sideways) plane the most. This makes it a particularly good exercise for strengthening the lateral stabilizers of the hip – the gluteus medius. If you perform this exercise well you will notice increased work in this outer hip muscle both on the supporting leg and on the moving leg.

Movement

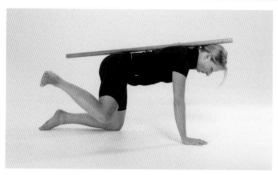

Drawing your belly button in to stabilize, and pushing down on the supporting hand and knee, slowly take your knee and opposite elbow out to the side, maintaining a right angle position at the knee and elbow. Only take your knee as far as you can without causing your hips to tilt, and as you move your arm outwards keep your elbow down and raise your upper arm by turning the thumb up (as shown). Your elbow should remain level with your hand to maximize the work in the rotator cuff muscles of the shoulder.

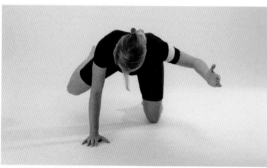

If your hips or shoulders tip sideways you have lost your alignment or gone too far into the position. The movement is not a very big one, but if you are doing it well, you will feel the work in the muscles at the sides of your hips and deep in your shoulders. Once you have gone as far as you can and maintained your core alignment, hold the position for 5 seconds, before lowering your arm and leg and changing sides.

How many reps and sets?

Perform 8–12 repetitions for 2–3 sets, with 30 seconds' rest between sets. Choose one of these exercises and work on it for 8–12 weeks before changing to another variation for best results. Alternatively, once you are familiar with all three variations you can do one set of each in order to get a *big bang* effect of stability in all planes of movement.

Abdominal strength in all planes of movement

In addition to avoiding too much flexion, it's really important to consider training your core in three dimensions, with both stability and movement in mind. Since we are designed to move in three dimensions off the bike, we need to be strong and stable in all planes of movement. On the bike we are predominantly moving and working in the sagittal plane – bending over to reach the bars, and bending and straightening our legs and hips within the pedalling action. The stability and strength demands are low, but it is often over longer periods or when pushing and pulling the bike from left to right standing out of the saddle, that stability and strength at the sides of the body and across the core in particular become important.

The exercises in this next section predominantly challenge the abdominal muscles but will also strengthen the surrounding core muscles of the hips and back, for a more stable centre with movements on and off the bike.

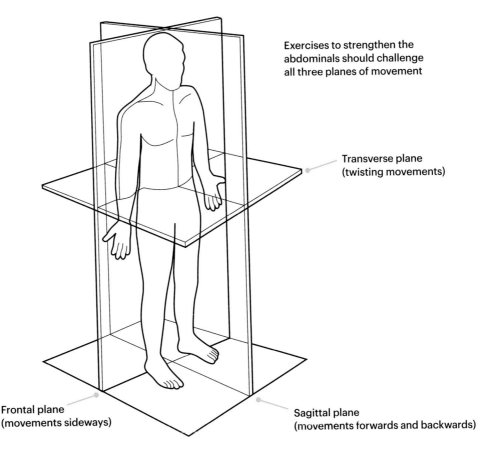

Exercises to strengthen the abdominals should challenge all three planes of movement

Transverse plane
(twisting movements)

Frontal plane
(movements sideways)

Sagittal plane
(movements forwards and backwards)

Exercises for sagittal plane core strength (forwards and backwards)

As cyclists we are moving mostly in the sagittal plane (forwards and backwards), but in a way not supportive of our innate design, and so our normal postural alignment and strength in this dimension is often negatively affected. For this reason, you may find that the exercises designed to challenge the core in the sagittal plane are the hardest to do well.

If in working through the exercises here you feel you can't do any of the variations with good form, don't worry. I simply suggest you leave them out altogether and come back to them at intervals to see if you are doing any better. Often, by working on the exercises in the frontal and transverse planes you will eventually break old habits and patterns that mean you can find good form in these exercises too.

Sticking to the form principle will help you change your muscle balance and alignment permanently as you progressively recycle these exercises into your programme design.

Whatever level you are working at, 'the form principle' must be applied consciously and consistently. The form principle dictates that you never compromise form for added load or difficulty. In other words, your position and your technique takes priority at all times. If you follow the technique points outlined in this chapter, and use the photos for guidance, you will achieve good form with the exercises here.

Planks

A plank is one of those exercises that can be great for core strength when done well, but actually diminishes core strength and can worsen muscle imbalances if done poorly. I have included a number of variations of the exercise here so that you have the best chance of choosing an option that can help you make a start on this exercise effectively. Some people favour the plank performed on the elbows, believing that it has more relevance to cyclists, particularly when resting on time trial bars. In my experience, cyclists are often more likely to perform a plank with poor form on their elbows, since the familiarity leads to the rounded shoulders of the flexed position on the bike. The 'forward ball roll' included here is an exception because it uses the instability of the moving ball to 'wake up' the core.

A good plank position strengthens the shoulders and upper back and is not meant to replicate the cycling position but correct for it, and a traditional plank on the hands opens up many more possibilities for classic conditioning exercises such as squat thrusts, burpees and press-ups.

If you find that your back aches in working through the plank variations here, or you are unable to maintain the alignment described, simply leave out the exercise altogether and keep coming back to it at intervals to see if you can do any better.

Swiss ball forward ball roll

The forward ball roll is my favoured variation on a plank for cyclists, as the instability of the ball in three dimensions gives you the best chance of stimulating the core to produce good alignment. The stable nature of the more traditional plank (on both the elbows and the hands) makes it all too easy for the cyclist's lazy body to drop into a poor position with inactive glutes, a dip in the lower back and often a rounding of the upper back. This ball version is a little more difficult to learn, but may give you the best chance of strengthening your lower abdominals and glutes in particular.

Preparation

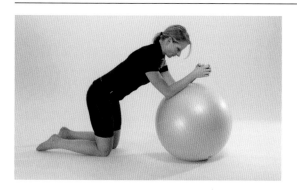

Start by kneeling behind the ball with your elbows resting on it, making a rectangular space underneath it into which you will then begin to move. Your elbows should be under your shoulders but slightly forwards, and your knees should be under your hips but slightly backwards, making a trapezius shape. Focus on a neutral alignment of your spine. You should have a natural curve at your lower back, and your hips, shoulders and ear should all be in line. Look down between your elbows to keep your neck in line. (The best way to learn this alignment is using the horse stance exercises already described.)

Movement

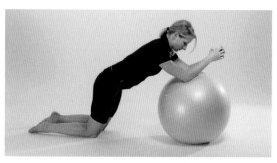

Draw your navel in and slowly move forward from the hips, opening up the angle between your thigh and your torso, maintaining the neutral alignment of your back. In practice this means tucking your hips under as you move forwards. You should feel your lower abdominal muscles and glutes working strongly. You should not feel this exercise in your lower back at all.

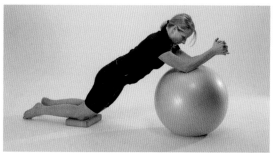

When you find a position that you can maintain, but feel that you are working the right areas, hold it for 5 seconds, before releasing backwards out of position. Sometimes it is difficult to get a feel for what your back position might look like, so positioning a mirror to one side, if at all possible, can help you connect what you see with what you feel.

Kneeling plank

Some cyclists will have a problem performing any plank with good form, but for others working into a full plank by first achieving good alignment in a kneeling plank can be the bridge that you need for the full version. Even if you are going to use the full plank as part of your core programme, I recommend going from the kneeling position first because I believe it's the best way to ensure you are doing the plank right.

Preparation and position

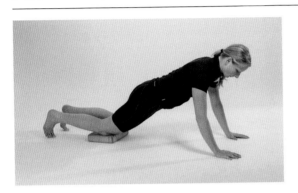

Kneel on all fours with your knees together, and if you have a hard floor, resting on a soft surface (Nichola, pictured, is using a yoga block). Keeping your hands positioned a little wider than shoulder width, walk your hands forwards while shifting your hips forwards and down. Keep moving in this direction until you are in the kneeling plank position shown, with your knees, hips, shoulders and ears all in one line.

Squeeze your thighs together, pull your tummy in, and squeeze your glutes. Your shoulders are softened away from your ears, and arms straight.

Plank on toes

Preparation and position

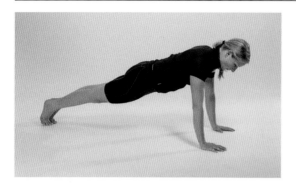

From the kneeling plank position, tuck your toes and push strongly through the balls of your feet, lifting your hips higher so that your ankles, hips, shoulders and ears are all in alignment. Squeeze your glutes together as you move, and brace yourself through your arms to support your body weight, but keep your elbows soft rather than locked.

Once you are in position, focus on squeezing your thighs together, pulling your tummy in at the front, and squeezing your glutes at the back. Keep your shoulders soft away from your ears and your arms straight but elbows not locked.

How many reps and sets?

Since this exercise is an isometric position, the focus is on increasing your core endurance in the position with progressively longer holds and shorter rest periods. In the set descriptions below, 'on' means that you are in the position and 'off' means that you come out of the position. Suggested progressions to work through are:

3 × 20 seconds on 10 seconds off × 2–3 sets

3 × 30 seconds on 15 seconds off × 2 sets

3 × 45 seconds on, 15 seconds off × 2 sets

3 × 1 minute held with 30 seconds' rest × 1 set

Though it may be tempting to go straight to the 'harder' sets here, it is more sensible to work through the progressions and focus on the quality of the position.

Swiss ball crunch

The Swiss ball crunch is the only type of 'crunchie' or 'sit-up' that I would recommend for cyclists, since the curve of the ball offers some support for the lower back as well as offering a counterbalancing backwards curve for extending the spine between sets.

The Swiss ball crunch does include some lumbar flexion so should be avoided by riders who have a history of lumbar disc injury. Good mobility in the upper back and a trouble-free neck are also prerequisites in order to include this exercise safely, so it may be better avoided if you know you have a very stiff upper back or any neck problem.

Preparation

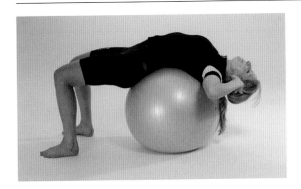

From a seated position on the ball, walk your feet forwards and lie backwards over it, keeping your weight over the ball as you go, until your back is curved around the ball and you are supported by it, but hanging slightly upside down as shown. You can vary how far back into this position you want to go by bringing your feet in closer (to push up and over more), or by taking your feet further away (and dropping your hips) to have a slightly less extreme start position. Your feet should be a little wider than hip-width apart to give you a stable base, and your knees should be directly over your ankles so that your shin is vertical. Rest your fingers by your temples (do not interlock them behind your head), with your elbows dropping out to the side.

Movement

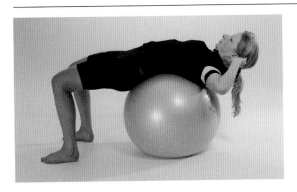

The Swiss ball crunch needs to start from both ends of your body, with a pelvic tuck at your tail end, and a chin tuck at your head end. The pelvic tuck ensures that your lower abdominals are included in the crunch while the chin tuck works the deep muscles of the neck that help to stabilize your neck.

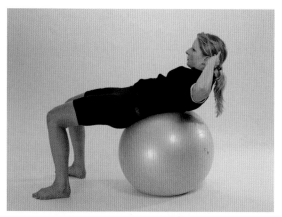

Initiate the movement with these 'tucking' actions, then continue to engage your abdominal muscles, until you feel your abdominals are fully contracted and there is no more movement. Note that there is not any actual 'sit-up' and the knee and ankle stay fixed through the crunch movement.

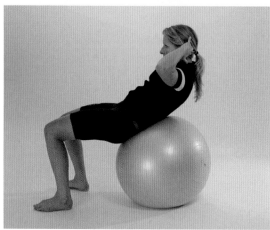

Pause briefly in this fully contracted position, before unravelling your body from the centre outwards in the reverse action, until you are fully extended over the ball in the start position.

(Neck crunch)

If you find that your neck hurts and is a limiting factor in this exercise, you can isolate the neck flexor muscles on their own to develop the strength to then be able to use your neck effectively in the Swiss ball crunch

Preparation

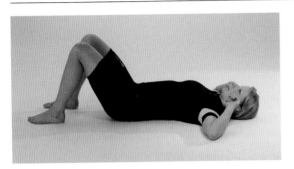

Lie flat on your back on the floor, with your knees bent as shown, and your fingers resting by your temples.

Movement

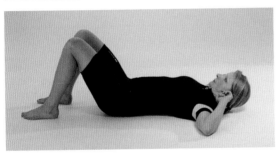

Keeping the back of your head in contact with the floor for as long as possible, lengthen the back of your neck to tuck your chin towards your chest, and lift the back of your head up off the floor by just a centimetre or two. If you are engaging your deep neck muscles effectively in this movement you should feel a throaty sensation as you engage the relevant muscles.

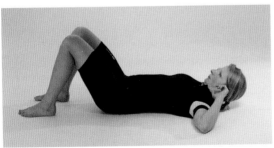

Lower your head back to the floor with control, keeping your chin tucked in and letting the back of your head touch the ground at the last minute.

How many reps and sets?

Perform 8–12 repetitions for 2–3 sets, with 30 seconds' rest between sets. Choose one of these exercises and work on it for 8–12 weeks before changing to another variation for best results. Alternatively, once you are familiar with all three variations you can do one set of each in order to get a *big bang* effect of stability in all planes of movement.

Exercises for frontal plane core strength (sideways)

Stability at the sides of your body is essential as the cycling action is unilateral, with a predominant downwards push on one leg at a time. Lateral core stability can help you maintain a solid centre as you push and pull alternately with the legs. Strength at the sides of your body becomes even more important when standing out of the saddle, climbing, or pushing harder when seated in the saddle.

The lateral gluteal muscles at the sides of your hips (the gluteus medius), the back muscles on either side of your spine, and the oblique abdominal muscles all stabilize against the force generated by the up-and-down movement of alternate legs. As the power you produce with your legs and hips increases, so must the stability and strength of your core muscles in the frontal plane.

Swiss ball side lean

This Swiss ball side lean exercise challenges all the muscles down the side of your body, from the lateral hip to the abdominals on one side and the muscles of the back on the same side. Building postural endurance in these muscles is important for standing climbing endurance in particular. With a stronger, more stable torso you will be able to stand out of the saddle for longer more comfortably. You will also be able to push harder for longer seated in the saddle.

Preparation

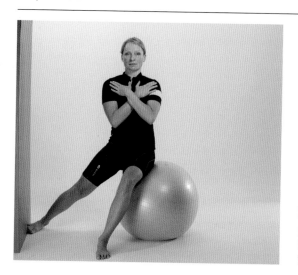

Sit sideways on your ball with your uppermost leg stretched out and braced against the wall, and the other leg bent and slightly forwards. Your feet should be a good distance apart to help give you a stable base of support for the lean. It's important you get a good anchor with the top leg so that you don't fall over the ball as you go into the lean. Position the ball so that you are sitting on half of the ball as you look down on it. Your hips and body should be facing forwards, perpendicular to the wall. Cross your arms over your chest and sit tall on the ball, drawing your navel in to prepare your abdominal muscles.

If you really struggle not to fall over when you get into position you can put both feet against the wall, spread wide but with your hips facing forward, as shown for the Swiss ball side bend that follows.

Movement

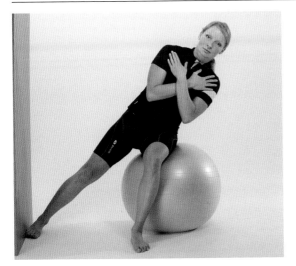

From this seated position, keep your navel drawn in as you lean over to the side, until your body is in line with your top leg making a diagonal. Your head and neck should be in line with your body, not tilting upwards, and with your chin tucked in so that your head is not forward of your body. Once in position, hold firmly, before bringing your shoulder towards your hip in a side bend to come back to a seated position on the ball.

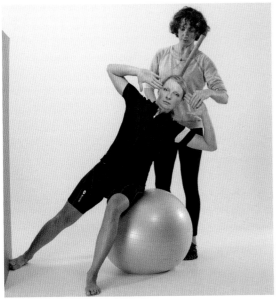

Here, I am using a dowel rod to check alignment in the frontal plane.

How many reps and sets?

Since this exercise is an isometric position, the focus is on increasing your core endurance in the position with progressively longer holds and shorter rest periods. In the set descriptions below 'on' means that you are in the position and 'off' means that you come out of the position. Suggested progressions to work through are:

3 × 20 seconds on 10 seconds off × 2–3 sets

3 × 30 seconds on 15 seconds off × 2 sets

3 × 45 seconds on, 15 seconds off × 2 sets

3 × 1 minute held with 30 seconds' rest × 1 set

One set of side leans means one set on both sides. Perform one side as described here, and then immediately the other.

Swiss ball side flexion

This side flexion exercise is a more dynamic version of the Swiss ball side lean. I highly recommend you work through the progressions of the side lean for several weeks before moving on to this Swiss ball side bend.

This exercise challenges all the muscles of the side body, but the dynamic movement develops the oblique abdominals in particular. This oblique strength gives you more power potential when you pull on the bars out of the saddle, to climb, to sprint or to accelerate uphill.

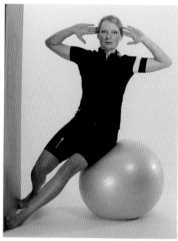

Preparation

Sit sideways on your ball with both legs stretched out and braced against the wall, as wide as feels comfortable and gives you a stable base from which to move. Position the ball so that you are sitting on half of the ball as you look down on it. Your hips and body should be facing forward, perpendicular to the wall. Hold your arms up, with your elbows out and your fingers by your temples. Sit tall on the ball, lifting your chest and drawing your navel in to prepare your abdominal muscles for the dynamic movement.

Movement

Bracing against the wall with your legs, keep your hips and body facing forward and bend over the ball until your elbow is lengthened across the ball, and then actively pull back in the opposite direction to side bend back to the seated position. This movement should be dynamic and springy, unlike the static side lean. You should take only a second to touch your elbow over the ball and bend back again. It is very challenging to move only in the sideways plane. Common technique faults can be: rotating your torso as you side bend, or slumping through your upper body. Work hard to keep your elbows wide, and your shoulder and hip in line throughout the movement to maintain good form.

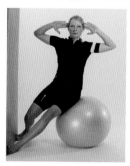

How many reps and sets?

Perform 8–12 repetitions for 2–3 sets. Switching sides saves time with this exercise, so it's best to work one side and then immediately the other side, with just a brief rest in between. One set of side bends means one set on both sides.

Exercises for transverse plane core strength (twisting)

Strength across your core is important on the bike when you stand out of the saddle, pushing with your legs and pulling on the bars as you move your bike from side to side underneath you. Core strength (and mobility) in a twisting movement is also important in maintaining a healthy spine and avoiding back injury. Loss of both mobility and core strength in a twisting movement can leave you vulnerable to back injury, more likely off the bike than on it, so working on your transverse plane core strength is an important preventative measure to include in your conditioning programme.

Swiss ball lower-body Russian twist

I have chosen this Swiss ball lower-body Russian twist because it's one of the safest ways you can start to strengthen your core muscles in a twist movement, even if you have a vulnerable back. It also helps to ensure that your inner muscles are working correctly and emphasizes the 'lower abdominals', which tend to be the weakest. It has the added benefit of helping to restore mobility at the same time, giving you a rotational stretch between every core contraction.

Preparation

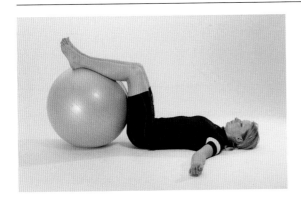

Lie on your back with your legs up on the ball and your arms out wide, palms turned up. Actively pull the ball close to you, so that it's hugging the back of your thighs.

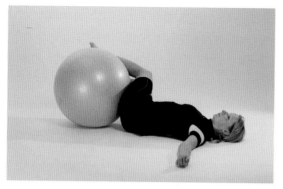

Keeping a hold on the ball by pulling it close, drop your knees to the right so that the ball rolls to the side. As your legs drop to the right, press down and back with your right arm so that you don't roll over, and catch the point when you can just keep your left shoulder on the floor.

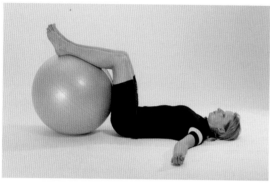

From here, draw your belly button in and pull the ball back to the centre, focusing on keeping the abdominals strong as you move.

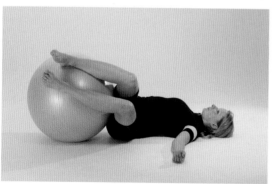

Then, drop your knees to your left so that the ball rolls to the side and repeat on this opposite side. Ideally, you should breathe in as you drop your legs to the side, and breathe out as you drag the ball back to the centre, drawing your navel in. This breathing rhythm should help you achieve the correct engagement of your deep core muscles.

Lower-body Russian twist with medicine ball

This variation with a medicine ball held between the knees is a simple and effective way to progress the exercise. The additional weight of the ball increases both the strength needed in the abdominal muscles, but also the range of the stretch.

Preparation

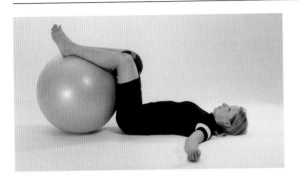

Lie on your back with your legs up on the Swiss ball, and your arms out wide, palms turned up. Actively pull the ball close to you, so that it's hugging the back of your thighs. Place a small medicine ball (2–3kg will be enough) between your knees and hold on to it by squeezing your knees together.

Movement

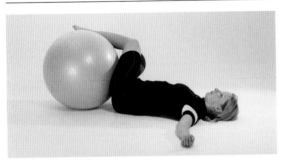

Stay in contact with the Swiss ball by drawing it close, and the medicine ball by squeezing your knees, drop your knees to the right. As your legs move, press down and back with your right arm so that you don't roll over, and catch the point when you can just keep your left shoulder on the floor.

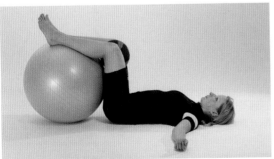

From here, draw your navel in and pull the ball back to the centre, focusing on drawing your belly button in as you go.

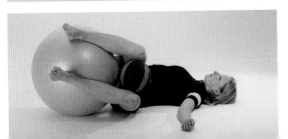

Then, drop your knees to your left so that the ball rolls to the side, and repeat on this opposite side. The breathing pattern is as for the previous exercise.

Swiss ball lower-body Russian twist with cross crunch

This variation of the exercise includes flexion at the end of the movement, and should be avoided if you have a history of lumbar disc injury or lower back problems. However, as a final progression of this sequence it allows for full contraction of the abdominal muscles in rotation at the end of the movement, as well as allowing you to progress from the basic exercise if you don't have a medicine ball.

Preparation

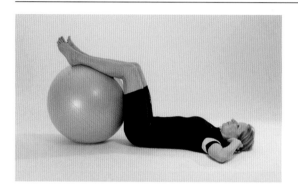

Lie on your back with your legs up on the ball, fingers at your temples and your elbows out wide as shown. Actively pull the ball close to you, hugging it with the back of Δyour thighs.

Movement

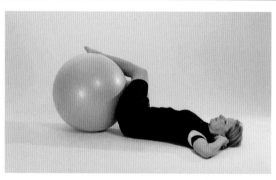

Drop your knees to the right. As you move, press down and back with your right elbow so that you don't roll over. Catch the point when you can only just keep your left elbow on the floor.

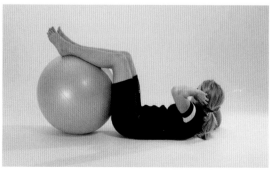

Draw your navel in and pull the ball back to the centre, curling up and bringing your left elbow across to your right knee. Your elbow does not need to reach your knee. Then release back, allowing your elbow to come back to the floor and your knees to drop to the side into a diagonal stretch. Breathe in as you drop your legs to the side, and breathe out as you drag the ball back to the centre, and 'cross-crunch' towards the opposite knee. This breathing rhythm should help you achieve the correct engagement of your deep core muscles.

Lower-body Russian twist with cross crunch (no ball variation)

If you have no Swiss ball available (for example if you are travelling) then you can perform this exercise effectively without any equipment at all. It helps if you have worked on the exercise variations with a Swiss ball first, but offers an equipment-free option if you need it.

Preparation

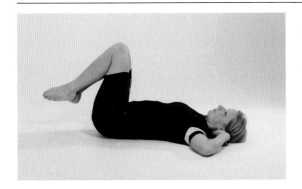

Lie on your back with your legs raised with your knees bent. Your knees should be directly above your hips. Rest your fingers at your temples with your elbows out wide, as shown. Actively engage your abdominals by pulling your navel in and imprinting your lower back into the floor.

Movement

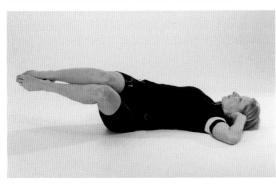

Keeping your core engaged, drop your knees to the left, keeping them perpendicular to your hips, and pressing firmly down with your left elbow so that you don't roll over. Catch the point when you can only just keep your right elbow on the floor, and then from here, pull your knees back to the centre, bringing your right elbow across to your right knee as you do so. Make sure that you feel your abdominal muscles are fully contracted (you need not 'sit up' so that your elbow reaches your knee), and then 'unwind' the movement, allowing your elbow to come back to the floor and your knees to drop to the side into a diagonal stretch.

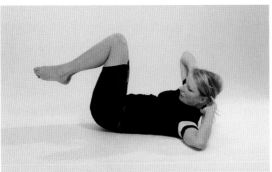

Breathe in as you drop your legs to the side, and bring both elbows to the floor, and breathe out as you drag your knees back to the centre, and 'cross-crunch' towards the opposite knee. This breathing rhythm should help you achieve the correct engagement of your deep core muscles.

Preparing the body for upright (axial) loading

This bicep curl is just one example of many simple lightweight dumbbell exercises that can be used to help train your standing postural alignment. As discussed earlier in this chapter, good standing posture is an important precursor to loading the body upright, such as with those exercises you will see in Chapter 3 on strength essentials. You can train the frontal plane by using one-sided exercises or the transverse plane by moving a dumbbell across the body or, as in this case with the bicep curl, target the sagittal plane by carrying weights in front of you.

Standing posture trainers (dumbbell bicep curl as an example)

Preparation

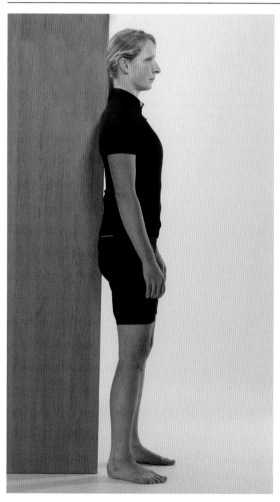

I recommend you use a doorframe for reference when you first try this exercise, or even throughout the exercise to give you some feedback as to how you are standing. Rest your back against a doorframe, with your feet about half your foot's length away from the door, and hip-width apart. Ideally you should be touching the doorframe in three places: your pelvis, between your shoulder blades and the back of your head. Bend your knees slightly and tilt your pelvis down at the back until there is a gap behind your lower back just wide enough for the thickness of your hand, but no bigger. Lift your chest and tuck your chin down to extend your spine and lengthen the back of your neck. If your thoracic spine is very stiff, you will struggle to make contact with the doorframe with your head. Don't force the position, but stand as tall as you can with your chin tucked down and the back of your neck long.

This position represents good upright posture and is what you are trying to maintain throughout the exercise. You can use the doorframe for reference in this way throughout, or try to adopt the same position without aid, by keeping soft knees, tucking your hips down slightly at the back, lifting your chest and tucking your chin down.

Movement

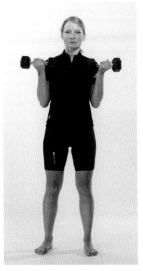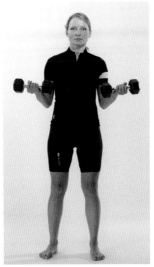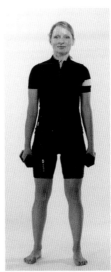

Adopting good upright posture and carrying two dumbbells at your sides, draw your navel in to brace your abdominals, and, keeping your body still, bend your elbows to raise the dumbbells to shoulder height. Pause in this position for a moment, before lowering them back to your sides with control. Try to keep your elbows tucked into your sides throughout and squeeze your shoulder blades together at the back, lifting your chest.

How many reps and sets?

Perform 8–12 repetitions for 2–3 sets, with 30 seconds' rest between sets.

Essential core
ready reference pictures

HIP AND LOWER BACK EXTENSIONS

Swiss ball hip extension feet on ball for gluteal and upper hamstrings strength

Arms out to sides

Arms across chest

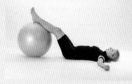
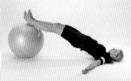
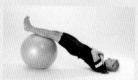

+ knee bend sequence

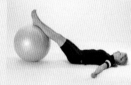
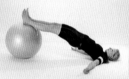
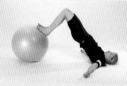
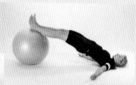

Prone cobra for improved upper back posture, strength and for a 'flatter' back on the bike

Off the floor

Swiss ball variation and Arms wide variation

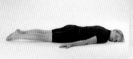
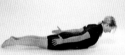
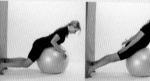

Alternating superman for rotational strength and flexibility in the back

Off the floor

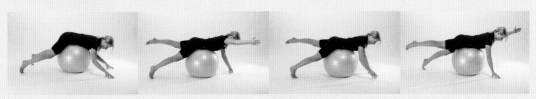

Swiss ball variation

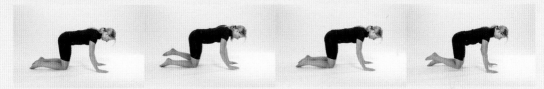

CORE WITHOUT FLEXION

Horse stances for 'inner unit' stability in three dimensions

Vertical

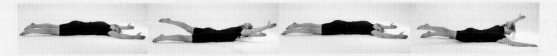

Working with a stick

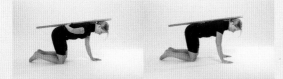

Horizontal   Abduction

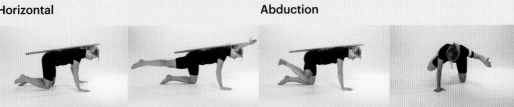

EXERCISES FOR SAGITTAL PLANES (forwards and backwards) abdominal strength

Planks

Swiss ball forward ball roll

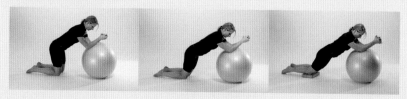

Kneeling plank   Full plank

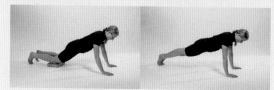

Swiss ball crunch (flexion with extension)

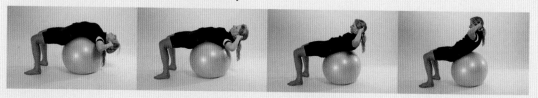

Neck crunch

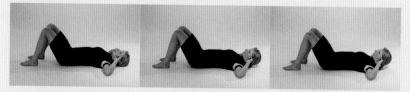

EXERCISES FOR FRONTAL PLANE ABDOMINAL STRENGTH

Swiss ball side lean

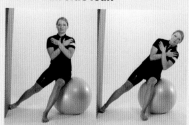

Swiss ball side flexion

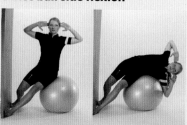

Swiss ball lower body Russian twist

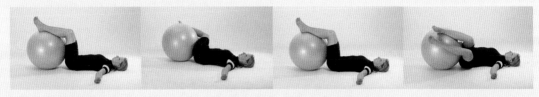

With medicine ball

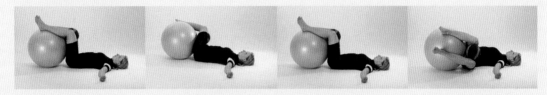

Swiss ball lower-body Russian twist with cross crunch

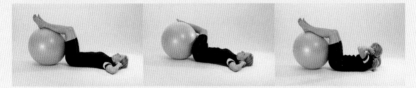

Lower-body Russian twist with cross crunch (no ball variation)

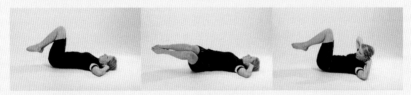

Standing posture trainers

DB bicep curl

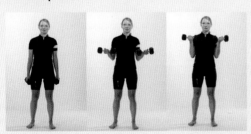

Using doorframe for reference

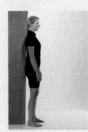

5. Cross-training

Overview of this chapter

What is cross-training?

Cross-training is the term given to using another sport or activity to improve your overall condition and physical fitness. For fitness enthusiasts, the goal will most likely be to have good 'all-round' fitness, but for cyclists the ultimate goal of crossing over to another sport is to bring back some valuable conditioning attributes to your cycling performance. Secondarily, and as important in the context of this book, cross-training can be a means by which cyclists maintain some of that all-important functional fitness that keeps you pain and injury free both on and off the bike, for a lifetime. With these dual goals in mind, in this chapter I am going to discuss the pros and cons of some of the main cross-training options most commonly used by cyclists.

Sometimes cross-training can be a pragmatic decision. You might be travelling without your bike and want to maintain some of your cardiovascular fitness and so use the hotel pool, or run on the treadmill. Or you might find that weather conditions outside force your bike training indoors, and so to get some fresh air and safe outdoor exercise you go for a short run twice a week, or play five-a-side football with your work colleagues.

Aside from the practical benefits, in this chapter I'm going to discuss the cross-training options that can actually enhance your cycling fitness in the long run, as well as help you stay injury free for the long term. At the end of this chapter you should be able to mindfully select those that are most appropriate for you, based on your current physical condition and the season relative to your cycling goals.

Choosing options that complement your conditioning

A common mistake with cross-training is to select activities that you are already good at, or that give you more of what you're already getting from your cycling training. A classic example might be choosing to participate in an indoor cycling class during the winter months to help maintain motivation and for cycling fitness.

'Spin' classes are good fun and can be great for general fitness, but they are often not ideal for cyclists for two reasons: Firstly, the position of most spin bikes is radically different from your actual bike set up, making it at the very least not all that specific to the cycling action, and at worst, provocative to any muscle imbalances or joint problems you may have.

Secondly, indoor cycling classes for the most part don't provide the structured training zone approach needed by most cyclists in their 'off' season. High-intensity intervals are often used to maintain interest and motivation within the group, and these tend to take your heart rate up and down throughout, without ever really settling on any consistent effort that might benefit your aerobic fitness. Consequently, you neither get the sport-specific adaptions that are most important in directly improving your cycling performance, nor do you benefit from other fitness components that are not so easy to obtain from your bike training, such as flexibility, stability or strength.

In introducing each of the cross-training options here, I will be encouraging you to choose those that give you some benefits across the spectrum of flexibility, stability and strength in particular, to complement the essential exercises I have worked through in this book from Chapters 2–4.

While some of the activities here challenge the cardiovascular system, and may therefore improve your aerobic fitness on the bike, as I discussed in more detail in Chapter 1, it is the sport-specific adaptions in both the central and peripheral cardiovascular systems as you work through the cycling movements that collectively give you your cycling fitness. In practice, this means that as a cyclist your aerobic fitness has to be developed as you ride your bike, unless you're unable to ride for any reason.

In some instances, particularly if you travel a lot, or if you live in an area where winter weather conditions are particularly harsh, you might consider the cardiovascular benefits of your cross-training options as more of a priority. For these reasons I will log the cardiovascular benefits for each activity so that if you need your cross-training choice to tick a lot of boxes in one go you can find something that will work for you.

Cross-training and the success formula

Once again in this chapter I will be referring to the all-important success formula, which helps you to hone your essential conditioning plan so that you are moving towards improved power potential and injury prevention, as well as a more balanced body all round. If you have been following this idea throughout this book, you will have some sense of where your priorities lie in terms of your own conditioning needs based on this formula.

Remember the success formula:

FLEXIBILITY
+ CORE STABILITY
+ STRENGTH
= **POWER POTENTIAL**

For each of the cross-training options discussed here, I will rate them on a three-star basis as having high, medium or low benefits for each of the main three areas of flexibility, strength and core discussed in this book. I will also rate the cardiovascular benefits out of three stars, in case this aspect is of particular importance because of frequent travel or unfavourable weather conditions giving you limited access to your bike.

No single activity can exclusively develop each aspect of your fitness without any benefits in other areas, and so gauging where each option fits in relation to what you want to get out of it will help you choose the best for you. If you prefer to work on your conditioning programme by yourself and would rather not include any of the cross-training methods discussed here, there is no need to include them as part of your plan.

In this chapter I will use a three-star system to rate the benefits of each activity in terms of flexibility, strength, core stability, and cardiovascular benefits. A score of three stars represents high benefits, a score of two stars represents medium benefits and a one-star rating represents low benefits. This three-star system should help you choose activities that complement the aspect of your conditioning that you are trying to develop at any given time, as well as helping you periodize your cross-training all year round.

Developing your biomotor abilities beyond the main three

Throughout this book I have focused on three key elements of conditioning: flexibility, strength and core stability. However, there are many other aspects to fitness in its broadest sense that I have not yet mentioned. One term used to describe these different elements of fitness is 'biomotor abilities'.

'Biomotor abilities' is a term used to describe how you move, relating in particular to the quality of the movement in consideration of a number of key physical attributes. Any activity or sport can be analysed in terms of its biomotor profile, to help you ensure that your training is specific enough for your body to adapt to meet the demands of the sport.

It is broadly understood that there are five main biomotor abilities, of which flexibility and strength are two, and co-ordination, endurance and speed are the other three. I consider core stability in the way I refer to it in this book to be a subgroup underpinning strength, and flexibility to be a sub-group underpinning optimal bike fit.

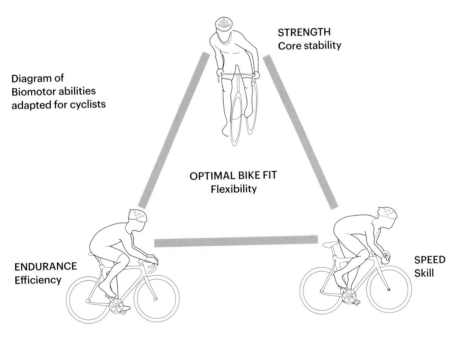

Diagram of Biomotor abilities adapted for cyclists

STRENGTH
Core stability

OPTIMAL BIKE FIT
Flexibility

ENDURANCE
Efficiency

SPEED
Skill

Endurance encompasses the cardiovascular elements that directly impact on your cycling performance and ability and may also be subdivided. While basic aerobic endurance is the main prerequisite upon which your cycling fitness is built, speed endurance and strength endurance are two subcategories that might be helpful in some circumstances. For example, a track cyclist would need these anaerobic fitness elements to allow them to continue to go hard without adequate rest or oxygen. They would also need greater agility, skill and coordination than most ordinary road cyclists to adapt to changing situations on the track, and to respond at the right time and in the right way. And there would be some carry-over between muscular strength and endurance strength, such that both are needed to maximize performance.

The introduction of different biomotor abilities when cross-training is one of the reasons it can be so beneficial for cyclists. Since the human body is dynamic and adaptive in nature, it will often respond well to a change in activity simply for the sake of change. Throughout this chapter I will explain any stand-out biomotor benefits in these broader terms too, to help you choose what's right for you.

Cross-training for injury prevention and rehab

Since cross-training often takes you into areas of fitness that are not explored through your cycling, there are some distinct physical benefits in terms of injury prevention. Overuse syndromes are common, particularly in straight-line endurance sports like cycling. The muscle imbalances that I describe in detail in Chapters 2 and 4 of this book in particular are often a precursor to injuries and issues. Where some muscles tend to get tight and others tend to become weak, joint health can begin to deteriorate, and with the high repetition of the pedalling action a change in emphasis can be a welcome break for the cyclist's body.

The saying 'a change is as good as a rest' is certainly one that helps explain the benefits of cross-training for cyclists. Where your body and mind can get bored with one activity, a change in focus can help open up new neuromuscular pathways that ultimately make you more capable when you come back to the bike. More than that, it can allow certain aspects of your fitness to take a 'rest' while you explore others.

Not only can cross-training help to prevent injury, but it can help you cope with injury too. For some cyclists, chronic injuries lead to periods spent off the bike, and for others crashes and the consequent fractures can lead them to seek out other activities to keep them sane. Most keen cyclists love being active, and when you can't ride your bike you will feel better for embracing the alternatives. What's more, when you can't ride, doing anything else that you can do safely will almost always get you back to fitness quicker than if you just wait it out doing nothing at all.

Psychological benefits of cross-training

As well as the physical benefits of cross-training, there are many psychological benefits. You can use cross-training activities to keep you motivated and interested in your training all year round, helping you to avoid the dip in motivation that is common if your cycling becomes relentless or monotonous. With any sport, the key to long-term improvements is consistency, and that means staying well, staying injury free as much as possible, and staying motivated. Many riders lose motivation because there is a lack of variety in their training, and for some a lack of periodization altogether. Periodizing your training both on and off the bike, and embracing some cross-training for variety, can be critical in keeping a plan progressing for long enough to see real gains in performance, well-being and even mood.

Periodization is the term given to the systematic planning of training in phases, with the goal being to achieve optimal performance for your main events in a season. Understanding how to build in some effective cross-training depends on creating differentiated training phases as part of your programme. The concept of periodization together with planning will be explained further in Chapter 6.

The mood-enhancing and social benefits of cross-training should not be underestimated, and for some cyclists for whom riding is largely a solitary pursuit, getting involved in a group activity can provide a much needed tonic that keeps you refreshed when you come to ride your bike solo. If you are a competitive cyclist, getting involved in a sport or activity outside of your cycling peer group can also help take the pressure off and avoid the performance comparisons that are often prevalent and sometimes depressing and demoralizing. Simply having some fun, and gaining some physical fitness as an added bonus, is a great way to fill some downtime or provide a welcome distraction when your cycling is not going as well as you would like it to.

Equally, if you know you are someone who prefers to exercise alone, or needs some quiet time to recover from a busy or hectic lifestyle, choosing a solitary pursuit or a more relaxing activity can give you what you need to keep your training on track from a holistic mind-body perspective.

Choosing cross-training activities that give you what you need psychologically is just as important as choosing them based on your physical needs. Knowing what works best for you from a mental-emotional perspective will help you to stay motivated and empowered throughout the training process, even when your cycling performance is taking a dip or you are recovering from injury. In this chapter I will encourage you to choose complementary cross-training options that suit you as a whole person, not just as a cyclist.

Seasonal considerations for your cross-training

Even if you are a recreational cyclist and not at all competitive, your cycling training should have some seasonal structure to help you work in training cycles that allow your body to adapt and improve. The same changes that help you to adapt for optimal cycling performance will also help avoid overuse injuries and issues caused by 'overtraining' any one aspect of your fitness to the detriment of the others.

'Variance' is a training principle that states that change must be an inherent part of a training programme in order for you to progress. Variance should take place across your cycling training as well as throughout your cross-training activities. Ideally, the changes that you implement for your cycling training should dovetail with and complement your off-the-bike conditioning.

Any training plan that does not change throughout the season will be ineffective in the long run and the same can be said of your cross-training activities too, that they should vary throughout the year so that you continue to adapt and respond.

For the most part, cross-training activities become more important in your 'off season', when you are spending less time on the bike, or working on your basic aerobic fitness, rather than pushing towards optimal cycling performance. A well-balanced, periodized off-the-bike conditioning programme should complement your cycling performance, as well as improve your all-round fitness as a functional human being.

The cross-training activities introduced here should be added to the essential conditioning elements that form the bulk of this book. They should be an optional adjunct to the exercises described in detail in Chapters 2–4, which should still form the main thrust of your off-the-bike programme. While selected stretch, strength and core exercises are crucial, complementing your efforts and adding variety and interest with cross-training can help you in the 'off season' in particular.

Problems associated with lack of variety and the benefits of cross-training

Symptoms of lack of variety

- Lack of consistency from season to season
- Prolonged periods without training, particularly at the end of the season when motivation is low
- Boredom, apathy, depression and poor lifestyle habits (such as overeating) at certain times of the year
- Recurrent 'overuse'-type injuries

Benefits of cross-training

- Consistency in training all year round, with a shift to include some cross-training in the 'off-season', or when necessary through injury or bad weather
- Good motivation and positive mood in relation to your exercise all year round
- Balanced lifestyle habits that support health as well as fitness
- Progression in performance both on and off the bike, year on year

Cross-training checklist

Good cross-training options for you should:
- Give you what you're not getting from the bike
- Respect where you sit on the success formula spectrum
- Fit in with your periodized training plan
- Suit your personality and mental, emotional and social needs
- Support a healthy lifestyle, as well as your cycling fitness
- Be fun and motivating

The Essential Conditioning Cross-Training Options

 Individual pursuits

Walking – making sure you put one foot in front of the other

Walking is the most fundamental of all movements, and as cyclists we sometimes have to remember to walk for health and well-being, instead of riding our bikes door to door from home to work, to school, to the pub or wherever. Ask most cyclists how much walking is in their day-to-day lives and it can be surprisingly little. If you're not sure how much you are glued to your saddle, then get yourself a simple pedometer and see how your stats stack up on a daily basis.

In Chapter 1 I described the evolutionary significance of our upright gait, and for the reasons described there I wholeheartedly believe that actively including some walking in your weekly schedule is essential for cyclists. At the most basic level, allowing a little more time to walk as part of your commute to and from work, or as part of your weekly routine can help to keep your joints healthy. Most importantly, walking gives your core and bones some stimulus via the ground forces that come up through your feet and ten minutes of uninterrupted brisk walking four or five times a week can be enough to keep you human.

Basic daily walking is essential, but I would not consider this kind of walking as part of your cross-training plan. I have mentioned it here because I know that many cyclists don't walk much at all. We complain when we stand on our feet for too long, and a shopping trip can become challenging for many of us in just a couple of hours. If this sounds rather too familiar to you, make an effort immediately to get more walking into your daily routine.

We all ought to know how to walk properly, but relearning to stand and walk with good posture is important if you want to maximize the benefits of the time you spend on your feet. Some of us need to remind our neuromuscular and musculoskeletal systems of what upright posture should look and feel like. Poor posture off the bike can be a significant problem for cyclists, especially as they get older, and the 'standing posture trainers' in Chapter 4 on core training should give you some pointers that you can use to give your walking added value by thinking about your alignment as you move.

Because efficient walking depends on an opposing arm and leg swing, it's worth ensuring that you're not carrying any heavy or awkward bags if possible anytime you are walking for more than a few minutes at a time. Poor postural habits can develop if you're carrying a bag on one shoulder, which will defeat the object of walking for improved posture.

Walking – as part of your cross-training

STAR RATINGS:

Flexibility: 1   Core stability: 2   Strength: 1   Cardiovascular fitness: 1–2

If you want to consider walking as part of your cross-training plan, then longer or more vigorous bouts of walking or hiking need to be part of your schedule. Walking briskly for 20 minutes or more, without carrying any bags, can help you focus on the rhythm of the movement. If you have a park or some off-road walking options nearby, walking on grass or woodland can add interest and variety of surface that can help stimulate your reflexes and keep you more alert in mind and body too. Hill repeats or step climbing can also be included where convenient to help increase the load through the muscles and joints and to increase the cardiovascular stimulus. If you find a steep hill locally that takes you between 30 seconds and a minute to stride up, then repeating that six to eight times can help strengthen the hips and leg muscles, as well as activating the core and benefitting the skeletal system.

For variety, or when the weather is too cold for cycling, longer hikes at the weekend can be an enjoyable way to get out in the fresh air. Be warned though, if you think you are fit because you are a cyclist, throwing a three, or four-hour hike (particularly if it's mountainous) into your programme on a whim may lead to significant muscle soreness or even joint injury, particularly around the knees or in the lower legs. Cycling does not encourage your body to work in the way that exercising on two feet does. It's important to approach these kinds of challenges by preparing

progressively, including brisk hill repeats, and stair climbing and descending in the few weeks leading up to any hiking adventures, to be sure you don't encounter any problems.

Running

Running is the cross-training option that most often trips cyclists up. The reason for this is that we are under the illusion that the fitness we have on the bike will count for something when we go to run. While it's true that both cycling and running stimulate the cardiovascular system and rely on endurance in the leg muscles, the musculoskeletal aspects of the two activities could not be more different. Cycling is very 'low-impact', negating ground forces altogether, allowing us to develop our aerobic fitness without developing any impact response to the joints or bones. Running is relatively high impact, with your body managing the deceleration forces involved every time your foot hits the ground, converting them into acceleration and momentum through the natural spring-like mechanisms of the muscles, bones and fascia.

Without question our bodies are designed to run, but whether we are fit to run depends on what our current status is in relation to the success formula.

In working through Chapters 2, 3 and 4 of this book, you will probably have some idea where you sit in terms of your overall condition off the bike. If you're very stiff and have a weak core, you're probably not in good enough shape to consider running as a cross-training option at this time. However, if you have been working on your essential conditioning for some time and have been including some of the functional strength exercises in Chapter 4, then some running may be a valuable and appropriate addition to your training plan. Even if this is the case, if you have not run or participated in any running games or athletic activities for some time, then I would approach running with caution.

The impact forces of running mean that you need to have good alignment, a functioning core, and no significant muscle imbalance issues in order to start to run without experiencing injury or problems.

Even if you know that your core works well, and your posture is good, take a measured and careful approach to introducing running so that you don't strain or sprain muscles or joints, or suffer from excessive muscle soreness that puts you off running ever again.

If you have a background in running or running sports, I would highly recommend you include a small amount of running as part of your off-season cross-training, as you will most likely be able to integrate some running relatively easily and without any problems. Bearing in mind the 'if you don't use it, you lose it' concept, you will find it much easier to maintain your running than start again from scratch some time in the future.

On a more positive note for beginners, if you are starting to run for the first time in a while, or for the first time ever, you have an ideal opportunity to establish good running form. Including short bouts of running or using running drills for technique can often be more effective than starting with slower, longer runs, which can lead to poor form, joint issues and injuries.

Consciously thinking about how you run, and running at a good speed for a given distance, before walking to recover, can be much better training. A football pitch in your nearest public park can be as good a place as any to start. Focus on running with an upright body, with good knee lift and driving with your arms, for the length of the pitch, then walk across the width of it before repeating along the other side. Three to six laps of this nature will be excellent running training for any cyclist.

Benefits of running

- Significant stimulus for the core muscles in particular
- The impact forces involved can improve bone density, strengthening bones, helping to prevent osteoporosis, and reducing the risk of fracture with falls from the bike
- Improved balance and agility, particularly if you include off-road running
- If you can run without issues, you can participate in many others sports, so that more cross-training options become open to you
- Combining the musculoskeletal benefits with cardiovascular fitness, and restoring our most human method of locomotion, running can be a good *big bang* cross-training activity, giving you lots of benefits in one go if you are travelling or short on time.

Risks of running

- If you run with muscle imbalances and a weak core, you are likely at risk of muscle or joint injury that may affect your cycling for some time
- Muscle soreness from running can be significant and long lasting if you do too much too soon, so a progressive introduction or reintroduction is prudent

How much is enough?

For most cyclists, introducing running as part of a cross-training session that includes other elements is a good way to begin to develop your running fitness without overdoing it. If you are doing some conditioning work at home, going outside to include some running at the start of your session can add interest and balance to a core- or strength-focused session. Always remember that the main benefits of running for you as a *cyclist* are those related to its impact nature, so just doing enough to stimulate some benefits without causing any problems will probably mean including at the most two bouts of perhaps 10–15 minutes per week as part of a core session, or for those with a background in running, one 20–30 minute run a week.

If you are including some running as part of a conditioning programme that has some stretching elements to it, include the pre-stretches before you go out to run as part of the warm up, and go straight into the strength and core aspects when you get back in.

Including short 10–15 minute runs as part of your essential plan can be a good way to experience the benefits of running. Perform any pre-stretches from your essential conditioning programme before you run and then any strength and core exercises after your run.

Treadmill running

For some cyclists who have access to a gym or sports centre, treadmill running may be an appealing option. However, treadmill running will not stimulate the natural biomechanical mechanisms of the body in the same way that running outside will. To point out the obvious, on a treadmill the ground is moving as you strike it, which makes the muscle recruitment and impact forces quite different to running on the ground. For these reasons, and in brief summary, I would not recommend treadmill running as an option for time-poor cyclists.

Footwear factors for cross-training in general

Minimalist footwear has become popularized in fitness and sports communities in recent years, and the ideology behind it dovetails well with the concepts I outline in this book. I would encourage you to use the most minimalist footwear that you can for all the essential exercises in this book through Chapters 2-4. By minimalist, I mean a shoe that is flat (rather than having a heel of any kind) and that has a relatively thin sole to allow you to feel the ground beneath you. In fact, if you are exercising at home, I would encourage you to work barefoot, since that is fundamentally how we are designed to function.

For running, I recommend you start on grass, which should help you work with a more minimalist running trainer. I'm not a fan of trainers designed with a big cushion under the heel to support the 'heel strike', when there is growing evidence that optimal running involves a mid-foot landing to facilitate the natural biomechanics of the foot, leg and all the mechanisms up through the body via the fascia.

A detailed discussion of footwear choice for running is outside the scope of this book, but I would encourage you to choose a more minimalist style trainer and start by running on grass, thus encouraging your body to develop a natural and efficient running style.

Swimming

STAR RATINGS:

Flexibility: 2–3   Core stability: 1–2   Strength: 1   Cardiovascular fitness: 1–2

For many cyclists, swimming is something that you either love or hate. For some, like myself, a general ability in endurance sports may mean that you swam to a good level when you were young, and have never really forgotten the skills and drills that you learned through length after length in the pool. Those cyclists who were first triathletes are also likely to be able to use swimming as an adjunct to their training with relative ease.

The other group of cyclists are probably poor swimmers, and find that when they do get in the pool one or two lengths can leave them so out of breath that the idea of constructively swimming for cross-training seems an impossibility.

In my view, both strong swimmers and weaker swimmers can use swimming as an effective cross-training option, provided you recognize what it can do for you, and use your time in the pool constructively and intelligently, rather than just thrashing out the lengths without much thought as to how you swim.

The biggest benefits associated with swimming are in improving flexibility and mobility, promoting relaxation and offering an alternative mode of exercise for injured riders who are forced off the bike. If you know you are very stiff and pick up injuries easily, swimming may be an ideal activity to add some variety to your conditioning plan.

If you have a fracture in your pelvis, hips or legs, or a serious enough soft-tissue injury that means you cannot ride or even walk easily, being able to embrace swimming as an exercise option can be what keeps you sane while you heal enough to get back on the bike.

There is both scientific and anecdotal evidence to suggest that exercising in the water does something special for your flexibility. The feel of the viscous fluid that surrounds you when you swim stimulates touch and pressure receptors around joints, which helps your body to loosen up and move more easily. Since water represents a very low-impact environment for movement, as well as supporting 90 per cent of your body's weight with its buoyancy, water-based exercise has been embraced in rehab settings for some time, enabling a quicker return to exercise and movement from injury.

The other unique thing about swimming, or any movement in water, is the resistance offered in all directions, which is of course a blessing and a curse when trying to move through it. The water surrounding you provides constant and immediate feedback. Learning to interpret the feel of the water and slip through it with the least effort is what makes the difference between a skilled and an unskilled swimmer.

Using drills and skills for variety and interest

Whether you are a good swimmer or not, since your main reason for being in the pool is to develop your flexibility, mobility and alignment, I would urge you to break down the time you have into distinct practices so that you are focused on efficient and effective movement that enhances these aspects from your time in the pool.

The simplest way to break up your time is by using all of the different strokes that you can swim in order to work your muscles and joints through the widest range of movements possible. An even better way would be to use drills and skills that focus on different elements of each stroke to maintain your interest and improve your swimming style.

The simple principle behind any drills and skills practice is to practise the whole stroke, then break it down into certain parts, before working on the whole once more. For the cyclist who is in the pool to improve their flexibility and mobility, this approach can not only make you a better swimmer but will also allow you to isolate certain joints and areas where you are looking for more mobility.

A very simple example might be to swim two lengths of front crawl, then swim two lengths of leg kick and arms only respectively, before swimming two lengths of front crawl again. If you have some swimming experience you may well remember certain practices and drills that you have used in the past that you could incorporate into your cross-training in this way. If you don't have much swimming experience, but plan to use swimming constructively in the off season, it might be worth paying for a swimming lesson with an instructor who can teach you some elements to work on to keep you motivated and engaged in what you are doing.

'Drills' as a term applied to exercise describes an element of the practice designed to focus on one aspect of a given movement or in a team sports context, the game. Swimming drills exaggerate or expose elements of the stroke so that you can work on them in a conscious way before incorporating them into your swimming style. Cycling drills can be used in the same way to improve your pedalling efficiency, for example by repeating a seated hill with an emphasis on using the up phase of the pedal stroke, in order to improve climbing style and efficiency while seated in the saddle.

Choosing strokes to suit you

Some swimming strokes are particularly beneficial for working on certain areas, while others can be problematic if you have specific postural issues that you need to work around. Contrary to what you might believe, the low-impact nature of swimming does not mean it's completely without problems in certain circumstances. For example, if you have neck problems, the hyperextended position of swimming breaststroke with your head out of the water can cause pain and worsen your problems. Equally, if you have instability issues in your lower back, or knee problems, you might find the hyperextension of the lower back together with the breaststroke kick to be problematic. In the section below I have broken down the three main swimming strokes into their benefits and potential issues for cyclists, so that you can choose what to include to give you the biggest benefits.

Front crawl

Front crawl is often the most difficult stroke for the inexpert swimmer (aside from butterfly) because of the timing and position needed when breathing. Although learning to breathe correctly can take some time and effort, once mastered, front crawl is a great option for cyclists looking to improve the mobility in their lower and upper back in extension and rotation. The crawling action of the arms (and counterrotation of the legs and hips) is much needed by those with a stiff thoracic spine, and the sideways turn of the head means that even with limited neck mobility you will be able to breathe and move relatively easily.

Even if you find the breathing part of front crawl difficult, I think it's worthwhile from a flexibility/mobility standpoint to swim front crawl as far as you can with your face in the water, and then stop to stand up when you need a breath before setting off again.

A simple push and glide off the wall, or off the floor of a shallow pool, represents a whole body stretch as you reach forwards with your arms and stretch your legs out behind you. This movement decompresses the spine and stretches all the muscles and tissues along the length of your body. The push and glide from the wall can be a drill in itself, which helps you develop this lengthened position, so don't be deterred from doing what you can just because your swimming is not to Olympic standards.

If you have a current shoulder impingement then swimming front crawl may not be recommended, as the extended arm position coupled with a stiff or rigid upper back can exaggerate the problem.

Backstroke/back crawl

If you are comfortable swimming on your back, it's well worth including some backstroke as it offers many of the benefits of the rotational action that come with front crawl without the difficulties associated with breathing.

In particular, backstroke will offer you the biggest benefits in terms of shoulder mobility, as the backwards rotation of the arms tends to stretch out the front of the shoulder, which can get stiff from hours spent on a bike.

Breaststroke

Although most people can swim breaststroke one way or another, swimming breaststroke with your head out of the water can lead to problems for the neck and lower back. The 'frog kick' leg action of breaststroke can also aggravate some knee problems, particularly if your leg kick is asymmetrical.

When swum correctly, breaststroke is an undulating, propulsive stroke where the head comes out of the water briefly for the breath and then is submerged again *at the same time as* the main thrust of the legs that propels the swimmer forward. The head and neck are lifted out of the water together with the upper body, allowing for an easy breath without excessive hyperextension of the neck, and the spine (and lower back in particular) is in a relatively neutral as force is generated with the propulsive phase of the leg kick.

In contrast, most casual breaststroke swimmers keep their head out of the water throughout all phases of the stroke, which leads to potential problems from hyperextension at the neck and lower back in particular, especially where the thoracic spine (or upper back) is relatively fixed in a hunched posture.

For these reasons, if you have neck problems and you swim breaststroke with your head out of the water, I would be cautious about including breaststroke swimming as part of your cross-training. Since the hyperextended position of your neck in the pool is very similar to your head and neck position on the bike, you may find that you provoke issues that might actually get in the way of your riding. Swim backstroke or front crawl with your face in the water as safe alternatives.

The breaststroke leg kick can be beneficial to cyclists because it strengthens the muscles of the hips and legs in the frontal plane, on the insides and outsides, as well as utilizing the glute muscles (where cyclists can often be weak) as prime movers in the action. The circular motion at the hip also can help maintain or improve hip mobility, balancing for the limited one-dimensional motion of the hip when pedalling.

Breaststroke leg kick practised on its own, with the arms outstretched in front and with your face in the water, is another drill that you can include for variety, and also to strengthen the glutes and leg muscles while at the same time mobilizing the hips.

Pre-stretching before swimming for maximizing mobility benefits

If the pool you are using is attached to a gym, you can maximize the flexibility benefits by including the essential pre-stretches that you have chosen from Chapter 2 of this book immediately before you swim. Mobilizing the spine in particular with the foam roller can prepare the spine for the movements in the water, and using pre-stretching and swimming together will give you a bigger benefit than using one or the other in isolation.

Benefits of swimming

- Improved flexibility and mobility in the spine, shoulders and hips in particular
- Using swimming drills and skills and swimming more than one stroke can help you personalize your swimming to maximize the benefits where you need them the most
- The low-impact nature of swimming makes it a relatively safe cross-training option if you have significant injury problems and issues that rule out some of the other alternatives
- The relaxation some people enjoy in the water, together with the focus afforded by practising drills, can have a beneficial mental effect, reducing stress and enhancing recovery

Risks of swimming

- Some strokes may be contraindicated for specific joint problems, in particular for some neck, shoulder, back and knee problems. Breaststroke swum with the head out of the water is usually the most provocative
- To get the most out of swimming as a mode of cross-training, you might need to upskill so that you can swim more than one stroke in more than one way

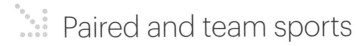

Paired and team sports

Indoor games and racket sports

STAR RATINGS:
Flexibility: 1   Core stability: 2   Strength: 1–2   Cardiovascular fitness: 2–3

Aside from straight line running, there are many team games in particular that offer excellent benefits for cyclists looking for a more social and varied cross-training activity. Indoor ball games such as five-a-side football (soccer), netball, basketball or any other indoor team game can provide some entertainment when the weather outside is at its worst, and when most cyclists are looking for off-season activities. Racket sports such as badminton, squash and (indoor) tennis are a few other options that might give you some of what you are looking for.

Not only do all of these sports offer some of the benefits discussed because of their running element, but since they require multidirectional movements they are also more likely to encourage the body to become active in three dimensions, through the natural inclusion of many of the primal patterns discussed in Chapter 1 and explained further in Chapter 3 on strength training. From a social standpoint, getting involved in a game with other players can be motivating and enjoyable too.

Stepping, lunging and twisting movement are elements included in all of these examples, which in particular are absent from cycling movements, and in broader terms the coordination and agility demands of games and racket sports are high too. Improving your reactions, balance and agility through playing games in the off season can help you apply these skills back on the bike in situations where you need to respond quickly to a changing situation.

In practice, it will be easiest for you to include these activities as part of your cross-training if you already have the skills needed to play the sport to a reasonable level. For example, if you played football to a good level at school or as a teenager, you are much more likely to be able to pick up a game of five-a-side and get involved without any issues. Deciding to play football if you have never really played before would be pointless since you will not have the prerequisites to get involved and reap the rewards, and also would be more likely to develop injuries and issues that would be associated with being a beginner and an adult.

In terms of the success formula, you probably need to have reasonable flexibility and core control, without any significant injury problems, to include games or racket sports for cross-training, although a high skill level in any sport (even if you haven't played for some time) will make it easy for you to get involved without any problems at a recreational level.

Benefits of indoor games and racket sports

- Multidirectional movement benefits, including some of the primal patterns (running, lunging, bending, twisting, pushing, pulling, squatting)
- Three-dimensional stimulation for the core muscles
- The impact forces involved have a positive impact on bone density, strengthening bones, helping to prevent osteoporosis and reducing the risk of fracture from falls from the bike (especially together with the below)
- Improved balance, agility, reactions and responses
- Indoor games and racket sports can have a completely different psychological focus to many cycling activities, which can be refreshing from a mental perspective
- 'Team' and 'social' benefits can maintain interest in exercise during the off season and enhance your mood and general well-being

Risks of games

- If you do not have a good level of skill in the sport as a foundation, you will be unable to get involved without the added risk of being a beginner
- Some team games have a contact element, which has an inherent risk of acute injury associated with it
- Muscle soreness from the multidirectional running element can be significant if you do too much too soon

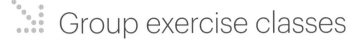

Group exercise classes

There are almost as many exercise class options as you can think of, depending on the current trends and on the exercise professionals operating in your area.

A group class of any kind is motivating and enjoyable because of the group dynamic, irrespective of how much interaction there is between participants. For the most part, when you go to a class you are exercising independently at the same time as other people. For some cyclists who often don't have the skills or background for team sports, this offers the benefits of being in a group without having to depend on your level of fitness or skill to participate.

In this section I am discussing three main classes of interest to cyclists that seem to have some longevity, but also are popular at the time of writing. Other options may be appealing and available to you, and I would encourage you to look at them through the same lens of evaluation I am using here.

Yoga

> **STAR RATINGS:**
>
> Flexibility: 2–3   Core stability: 2–3   Strength: 2   Cardiovascular fitness: 1

I am introducing yoga in its broadest sense, from my viewpoint as a cyclist first, and exercise professional and sometimes participant second. I am acutely aware that traditionally yoga has spiritual practice and mindfulness at its heart, but for the purposes of the cross-training discussion in this book I am mostly evaluating it in simplified, physical terms.

That being said, the first thing to know about yoga is that there are many different styles, and where one might not suit you at all, another might give you exactly what you are looking for. Some styles of yoga are very dynamic, involving standing poses and postures that combine a strong contraction in some muscles with a stretch in the opposing muscles, and with the core being active throughout. The whole-body engagement of standing poses combines many of the primal patterns that I have discussed throughout this book in combination (lunging, squatting, bending, twisting, pushing and pulling), using your own body weight for load, and often holding the positions for progressively longer periods to develop muscle strength and postural endurance.

Many styles of yoga include a strong balancing component too, with single-leg exercises and movements that most cyclists will find difficult to start with, but which for exactly this reason can offer significant benefits if you persevere. Yoga 'flow' sequences combine strength and balance components woven together in a chain of movements which is repeated several times over as you stretch and strengthen your way into a better position, and as your body warms up.

Other styles of yoga again can be more passive in nature, using floor-based positions and a focus on breathing to relax and let go of any tension, bringing about a progressive stretch in certain areas by using your body weight and the position to release the tension. Mindful deep breathing and relaxation may be a more prominent aspect, offering a more regenerating and meditative feel to a class, which for the most part gives the impression of aiding and enhancing recovery rather than expending energy in the process of the practice.

When most cyclists turn to yoga for cross-training they think of its flexibility benefits as the main attraction, but the many different styles and types of yoga mean that different attributes of fitness will become more prominent depending on the class you have chosen. Some styles emphasize strength and balance through standing postures, or flow sequences, while others emphasize breathing and relaxation through floor-based stretches. Trying out a number of classes before finding the style that suits you the best is highly recommended.

In practice, some yoga styles can be quite difficult to grasp for cyclists who don't have an athletic or gymnastic background, so choosing the right class that gives you what you need can be really important.

Even more important, in my view, than finding the right style of yoga is having a good instructor who will help you achieve a good position, using the right muscles in the correct way. Many of the positions are relatively complex compared to the essential exercises I have included in this book, and so having an instructor direct you into the right place so that you share the load effectively is particularly important.

Everyone has to start somewhere, and any good class instructor will offer various levels of an exercise to encourage you to get the most out of each movement or pose in a safe and appropriate way for your level. Pay close attention to what you are told to do, and expect to work hard both mentally and physically, and you will find that your understanding and ability in yoga will improve the more you attend class.

As with many of the cross-training options discussed here, but particularly with any form of group exercise, I would recommend you commit to the same class and instructor on a weekly basis for 2–3 months at a time. This allows you time to understand what you are doing and physically adapt to the exercises.

With something like yoga, an occasional intermittent class is unlikely to be sufficient for you to progress and develop your practice enough to grasp even the basics. Most cyclists will find yoga difficult because the skills and conditioning elements involved are outside your abilities at the outset. Rather than dismissing yoga as a result, if you remember that the whole purpose of cross-training is to work on your weaknesses you might find that the rewards are surprising.

Yoga and hypermobility

If you are hypermobile, yoga may seem particularly attractive because, compared to your cycling peers, you seem to be quite good at it at the first attempt. However, if you're hypermobile and want to include some yoga as part of your cross-training, you need to be more careful to choose the right kind of yoga for you, and a good instructor. On the face of it you will seem to be more flexible and more able to achieve positions and poses, but there is a risk that without proper preparation you may be 'hanging' and 'hinging' off hypermobile joints. For this reason, the more dynamic or 'stronger' yoga styles will be more appropriate for you, and with good instruction you will be taught to use your muscles to actively engage with the poses, rather than passively drop into them.

Benefits of yoga

- Potentially wide-ranging benefits, including improved strength and flexibility, balance and coordination, as well as relaxation and many far-reaching benefits associated with deep breathing
- The varied types and styles of yoga classes available means that you are likely to find one that you enjoy and benefit from if you take the time to find one that suits you

- The relaxation, mindfulness and meditative nature of some forms of yoga can help enhance recovery both physically and mentally

Risks of yoga

- For some hypermobile individuals, poor technique in a yoga class can lead to injuries associated with stretching joints and their surrounding tissues rather than muscles
- Muscle soreness from some of the deep stretching and strengthening that can happen in yoga can be significant while you adapt to the style of exercise

Pilates

STAR RATINGS:

Flexibility: 1–2   Core stability: 3   Strength: 1–2   Cardiovascular fitness: 1

Pilates as a system of exercise has evolved significantly from its original roots devised by Joseph Pilates in the early 20th century. As a physical culturalist, Pilates believed in the importance of mindful, conscious movement in maintaining a healthy physical body, and anticipated the impact that modern lifestyles were to have on people's health and well-being well ahead of his time.

Modern Pilates has developed in a number of different directions, but most classes still hold true to the original principles of concentration, control, centring, efficiency of movement, precision and breathing. For cyclists, the emphasis on alignment, core control and body balance is very complementary to many of the elements discussed in this book, and Chapter 4 on core essentials in particular.

As a cyclist you may have access to two types of Pilates, the more mainstream style that you will come across in a fitness environment, and the more 'clinical' Pilates that you may encounter in a rehab setting.

Many physiotherapists are trained in clinical Pilates which focuses more closely on correct engagement of deeper 'inner unit' core muscles that are often implicated in back pain, but also knee and hip problems. If you have been to a physiotherapist for treatment of one of these problems, chances are your rehab exercises may have included some Pilates.

The key concept in Pilates which defines it as separate to other systems of exercise is the idea of body control coming from the centre. In general, Pilates movements are slow and relatively isolated. Some of the movements may seem minimal, with a focus the quality of that movement more than the range or extent of the movement itself. In a Pilates class there will be distinct instructions on how and when to breathe, and how and when to engage your deep abdominal muscles in particular.

In Chapter 4 of this book on essential core exercises I gave you an overview of how the 'inner' and 'outer' abdominal muscles should work to provide both stability and strength to your core, and in Pilates you will find a good deal of emphasis on the inner muscles in particular.

If you are looking for a Pilates class in a fitness setting, often the class will begin with some standing work before moving on to the 'mat work', which is performed on the floor. Standing postural work led by an instructor can be particularly beneficial in helping cyclists become aware of their alignment, and in learning to correct it. The mat work is divided into exercises on all fours (some of which have some overlap with the 'horse stances' I introduced in Chapter 4), exercises lying on your side, and on your front and back. The mat work is designed to isolate areas around your core in three dimensions.

Clinical Pilates classes are more likely to be taught by a physiotherapist in smaller groups, with more personal attention to form and correct core engagement given by the instructor. Often these classes are exclusively focused on the mat work in order that correct engagement is learned in an isolated way, before moving to standing exercise variations. If you have been referred to a clinical Pilates class by a physiotherapist, it would probably be wise to attend in order that you learn correct technique before moving into a bigger class in a fitness environment.

One of the biggest challenges to cyclists attending a Pilates class is understanding what it is you are supposed to be doing. A common first experience is to come away feeling like you weren't 'doing anything', and therefore could not see how the class could benefit your fitness in any way. I must confess that this was my first experience too, even though I have subsequently trained in clinical Pilates techniques as part of my work.

In a way, if this is your experience you can be sure that you have a lot to learn from Pilates and that if you engage with the problem you will start to see the benefits. Patience is not a strong point for most cyclists who prefer the simplicity of repetitive pedalling. However, perseverance should mean that you gradually understand the workings of the class as well as your body.

Some Pilates classes may leave you coming away feeling better in yourself, perhaps slightly more flexible, or a little bit taller, in spite of the fact that you didn't really feel that you were doing very much. Generalized muscle soreness is rare in response to Pilates, and the place you might feel that you have been worked is often in and around your core.

Benefits of Pilates

- A clear and direct focus on core control and alignment offers huge benefits for most cyclists
- Support from an instructor to help you engage your deeper or inner abdominal muscles correctly can pay dividends when tackling other conditioning exercises (such as those in Chapter 4 of this book)
- Isolated, focused exercises where movement is slow and deliberate can be easier to follow for cyclists whose overall movement skill can be low
- Increased body awareness and control means improved movement all round
- The impact of Pilates can often be quite subtle, such that a Pilates class will be less likely to leave you with muscle soreness that will impact your cycling training
- Pilates (and clinical Pilates in particular) is a very safe form of exercise, even if you are in rehab from an injury

Risks (difficulties) of Pilates

- Pilates can be slow, and requires patience and determination to understand the movements and execute them correctly
- Without regular practice and a good instructor, you may not get the hang of what you are supposed to be doing, and so some of the potential benefits may elude you
- Some Pilates classes may include a lot of flexion exercises (such as sit-ups from the floor), which may be provocative for some cyclists who have lower back problems in particular.

Circuit training

Of all the options discussed in this chapter, circuit training has the *biggest bang* of potential benefits from one session in one hit.

A circuit of exercises can comprise any number or type of exercises, which are repeated for either a given number of repetitions or a set amount of time. Traditionally, a circuit will be largely made up of body-weight movements that stimulate both cardiovascular fitness and muscular endurance at the same time.

Many of the primal patterns discussed throughout this book and in Chapter 3 in particular, including lunges, squats, jumps, stepping exercises and shuttle runs, are likely to be included as part of the circuit. Often more core-focused exercises such as press-ups, squat thrusts, back extensions and sit-ups are also part of the workout.

Instructor-led circuits can be found in fitness clubs and in sports clubs, and some cycling clubs may offer a coach-led circuit as part of their winter training. While the instructor or coach is there to teach technique and manage the timings of moving from one exercise to the next, typically their main role is in motivation. Traditional circuits are tough and intense, pushing you into anaerobic territory where you will be breathing hard and feeling progressive muscular fatigue and lactic acid build-up the longer the circuit goes on.

While circuit training offers so many potential positives, it can also be problematic for cyclists for a number of reasons. Firstly, good technique in some of the body-weight and core exercises listed here are a prerequisite to being able to maintain your form for prolonged sets and multiple circuits. For example, if you cannot perform a good press-up in its own right, you certainly won't be able to maintain a good press-up for a minute or two at a time, as you might be asked to in a group session. Secondly, some of the running and jumping elements designed to raise the heart rate may be cause for potential injury for cyclists who are deconditioned in dealing with ground forces and can't handle running without problems.

As with any group class, alternative levels of the exercise can be offered and suggested by an experienced instructor so that you can maintain good form throughout, or alternatively you will be encouraged to switch to an easier version of the exercise as you fatigue. If you continue the exercises with poor form, the template that your body will remember as a movement pattern for that exercise will become 'bad habit', which can be much harder to break than starting from scratch with a new exercise.

Once again, the responsibility falls to the coach or instructor leading the circuit to ensure that while motivating and pushing the participants, he or she ensures that form does not suffer to the extent that either injury risk increases, or that a poor pattern may become learned. In some cases, this may mean the intensity of the workout may be required to drop off in order to ensure that movement technique is not compromised. Patience and a longer-term view might be required by both participants and coach in order for cyclists to develop the condition needed to get both the aerobic and muscular benefits available with a circuit training class.

In spite of these difficulties, I believe instructor-led circuit training is one of the best 'old school' methods for maintaining, or even improving fitness in a cyclist's off season, and if combined with an individual essential conditioning programme comprising the exercises in this book, you could find that year on year your ability to perform the body-weight basics that make up a traditional circuit improves dramatically.

Benefits of circuit training

- Traditional circuit training potentially offers the biggest cross-training benefits of all the activities discussed here, including body-weight strength through many of the primal patterns, focused core-strength exercises, and running elements that raise the heart rate
- The running and jumping drills that are often included have a positive impact on bone density, strengthening bones and helping to prevent osteoporosis
- The core elements can help improve and maintain alignment and posture
- Rapidly moving from one exercise to the next can improve agility, balance and athleticism

- The potential anaerobic element of a traditional circuit can be enjoyable and motivating in the off season, when most cyclists will be working at lower intensities or more steady-state types of training
- Combining the cardiovascular fitness, body-weight and core-strength benefits, a traditional circuit can be a *big bang* activity, giving you lots of gains in the minimal time

Risks of circuit training

- Performing many of the exercises included in a traditional circuit requires mastery of certain body-weight basics as a prerequisite
- The fatigue that is induced by the prolonged sets and repeated circuits can lead to poor form, which may in turn lead to bad movement habits if left unchecked by an instructor
- To get the most out of a circuit and achieve its *big bang* benefits may require some patience and a longer-term approach to your cross-training, including season-on-season progression through the conditioning essentials in this book in order that you reach a level of competency where circuits are all that they can be

6. Periodization and planning

 Overview of this chapter

MAKING A SEASONAL PLAN (page 259)

» Autumn (post-season)

» Winter (off season)

» Spring (preseason)

» Summer (in season)

» Typical seasonal schedule and adaptations

» Remembering the success formula – personalizing your approach

» Reviewing your seasonal plan

MAKING A WEEKLY PLAN (page 269)

» Example weekly review

» *Your* typical week of cycling, life and conditioning time

» Where to place key cross-training activities

» Using time-based templates to design your own conditioning programme

» Using the conditioning templates

THE ESSENTIAL CONDITIONING TEMPLATES (page 275)

» 10-minute templates

» 20-minute templates

» 30-minute templates

» 40-minute templates

What is periodization?

Periodization is the term given to the systematic planning of training in phases, the goal being to achieve optimal performance for your main events in a season. In physiological terms, a periodized training plan takes advantage of the body's stress-response mechanisms, which allow for progressive improvements in performance by adapting to the changing demands of structured training.

A good training plan will allow enough time for the body to adapt to the training load of any given session or set of sessions, and then change the training stimulus before the body becomes exhausted from overexposure to that same training.

Physical fitness of any kind is developed by way of this stress-response mechanism, which was first outlined by endocrinologist Hans Selye in the 1950s. His general adaption syndrome (GAS) model was subsequently developed further by exercise physiologists and sports coaches in the 1950s and 1960s to form the foundation of the science of periodization that sport scientists use today.

The science behind periodization and planning can be quite complex, but by simplifying the main elements and working to a basic plan you will find that you progress from one month to the next with purpose and clarity, and from season to season with more consistency than working without a time-scaled plan.

General Adaptation Syndrome

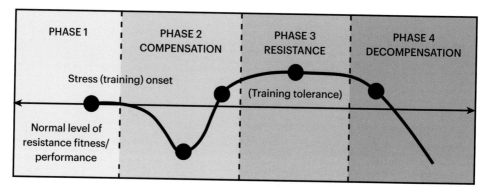

Separating your training into cycles

In addition to understanding the basic tenets of the stress response, the other key aspect of periodization that will help you the most is breaking your plan down into separate training cycles. Traditionally, a training plan is split into blocks so that you work backwards from your main goal event. For most cyclists the biggest 'chunk' of time to consider in planning terms would be the forthcoming year, which would be called the *macro*cycle. For Olympians the macrocycle might be even bigger, representing the four-year cycle between Olympic games.

In this chapter I will be encouraging you to think big first, taking a view of your next year of exercise in the context of what you did last year, and what you hope to do the year after that. Although you are (probably) not an Olympic athlete, one of the main reasons for lack of progress from one season to the next is this lack of perspective. Taking your sport and fitness goals and placing them in the context of your life in general can also give your training longevity, ensuring the consistency that is needed to maintain your health and fitness for the longer term so that you maximize your performance potential.

For most sports people, the intermediate amount of time to consider in your training plan would be a month or six weeks, and this would be called a *meso*cycle. In this chapter I will encourage you to develop your own mesocycle plan based on the four seasons so that each plan will be three months (or 12 weeks), with room for a slight change or progression at the halfway stage.

The smallest chunk of time to consider in your training plan is called a *micro*cycle, and for most people this would be a week. Towards the end of this chapter I will encourage you to get specific about what a week's training should look like for the current phase that you are in. For most people who work a 9–5 job, a weekly plan can be consistent and fairly structured. For others who have more varied work patterns, a weekly plan may consist of a menu of training options that can be fitted into the schedule with a little more flexibility. A plan does not have to be completely rigid to work, but needs to have some overarching goals and structure.

Why is planning so important, even for keen amateurs?

You might be thinking at this point that this all sounds a bit *serious* and technical for you and what you are looking to achieve, but I assure you it's not.

Most of you have probably heard the cliché 'If you fail to plan, you plan to fail', but like many sayings that have stuck, there is a lot of truth in this statement.

If you expect to get better at cycling just by riding your bike more, you are likely to plateau very quickly. It's true that if you are unfit you will see a steep improvement at the beginning, but it won't be long before you find that your fitness seems to be staying the same at best, or in some cases actually starting to get worse. If anything, your conditioning plan is more complicated than your cycling training, since you are looking to correct and balance for the time you spend on the bike, as well as ensure you are working through the elements of flexibility, strength and core detailed in Chapters 2–4.

Taking time out to plan your training, even in the simplest way, can make an enormous difference to how you feel about your cycling as well as your conditioning programme. Deciding what you want from your sport and making a plan to go after it can be a very empowering experience, and the learning that goes with getting to know what your body wants and needs can put you in a strong position to coach yourself on your journey towards better performance as well as health and fitness.

In my view, the time you spend on planning your programme is the most important of all, since once you have a plan, you simply have to get on with it, without needing to think about it for several months at a time.

Furthermore, if you take a more medium- to long-term view of planning your training, it makes it easier for you to factor in changes that accommodate whatever else is going on in your life, such as career or family commitments, moving house or any other personal matters that need to take priority at any given time. Rather than ignore these more holistic aspects relating to your performance, by planning to allow for that change and structuring your training to accommodate it you can often come back to full fitness with renewed vigour when the time comes.

Dovetailing your conditioning plan with your cycling training to progress with both

In this chapter I will be focused on helping you develop the detail of your essential conditioning plan off the bike using the exercises in this book. The periodization of your conditioning should be connected to and balanced by your training on the bike, so I will be offering some very broad ideas about your cycling plan too.

It is outside the scope of this book to look in any detail at the periodization and planning of your sport-specific cycling training. Much has been written about cycling training and if you don't already have some broad ideas about what aspects of your cycling fitness you should be developing and when, I would urge you to look out some resources that will help you, or seek out a cycling coach.

If you already have a cycling training plan, or have a coach who helps you with your training, the planning of your conditioning programme to complement that should be even easier. The more awareness you have about what you will be doing on your bike and when, the easier it will be to slot in some appropriate conditioning.

Many of the problems associated with a lack of cross-training or conditioning in your programme are inherently connected with a lack of planning and periodization, so you will see many similarities here to the 'problems and benefits' list in Chapter 5 on cross-training.

I believe that for many cyclists a periodized conditioning plan is the missing piece in the puzzle that strings seasons together, giving you sustainable and improved performance and a better sense of health and well-being all round.

Problems associated with a lack of planning and periodization

- Lack of consistency in cycling performance from season to season
- A progressive decline in your overall condition off the bike, leading to niggles and injuries and issues that sometimes take years to develop
- Prolonged periods without regular training or exercise, either through low motivation or because of chronic injuries and progressive muscle imbalances
- Boredom, apathy, depression and poor lifestyle habits (such as overeating) at certain times of the year associated with a lack of structure and purpose

Benefits of developing a plan

- Consistency in training all year round, and from one year to the next
- A robust body, both on and off the bike, that allows you to do what you want to do
- Plenty of variety due to seasonal variations, and the dovetailing of cycling training with off-the-bike conditioning and cross-training
- Good motivation and positive mood in relation to your exercise all year round
- Balanced lifestyle habits that support health as well as fitness
- Progression in performance both on and off the bike, year on year

General planning guidelines

Motivational factors

Much has been written about goal setting that you can find with an easy google search, so I need not go into great detail here. The SMART acronym is a good summary of where to start with your goals before we broaden the discussion further.

Smart goals are:

Specific • **M**easurable • **A**ttainable • **R**ecorded • **T**ime bound

Many recreational sports people believe that a legitimate goal to be working towards has to be a performance goal, such as achieving a particular time in a time trial, or a certain placing in a given event. But in the broader context of cycling for fitness, or conditioning for health, process goals are very important, and may even be the only type of goal that you need to use to structure your training. I have found that goals relating to being more consistent with training of any kind are extremely important in building momentum that leads to better performance. You may simply set yourself a target of cycling four times a week, or for two hours on both days at the weekend, or of stretching for 10 minutes every evening, and then log your progress for a given period so that you can evaluate how you have done at the end of it.

A process goal is one that deals with the training detail that leads to better performance by default, rather than focusing on the desired performance itself. For many cyclists I have worked with of all abilities, a focus on processes can maintain motivation by way of seeing clear and direct achievements in a particular skill or ability to consistently perform an exercise.

In the context of conditioning examples, if you know that you are stiff and would like to be more flexible, then you probably realize that regular stretching will get you to that desired goal. You can make that goal SMART quite easily by using the exercises in this book and by simply putting a stretching plan together.

For example:

- You can set the goal to become more flexible in your hamstrings at the knee (that's specific – S).
- You can measure the improvement in your flexibility by working through the supine hamstring stretch as shown in Chapter 2 (the higher you are able to raise your leg, the more flexible you are becoming – M).
- You can be confident that the goal is attainable (because I have selected stretches here that I know are effective for cyclists – A).
- Commit to the conditioning exercises that relate to your flexibility goals, and write them down as part of your exercise plan (that's recorded – R)
- And you will work on the same programme for a period of three months, to allow your body time to adapt and change (that's time bound – T).

That wasn't too complicated, was it. That's SMART conditioning.

If you are unclear what your cycling goals are at this stage, don't panic. Even if all you know is roughly the amount of cycling you want to do at different stages of the year, you can dovetail some conditioning around that riding to develop your functional fitness and cycling potential. You can use the natural cycles of the seasons to ensure that you are working through a range of stretch, strength and core work to support your bike riding, and allow for that better cycling performance when you are ready to commit in more detail.

Writing something down and being accountable

Perhaps the most important letter of the SMART acronym for me is the R, Recorded. In SMART goals the R usually stands for Realistic, and for me that's about making a record to stick to. There is something about writing down your plan, or even sketching out some ideas that takes it into the action stage by committing it to paper.

In this chapter I have included various planning templates that you can photocopy and scribble over as many times as you like as you create and change your plan through the seasons. I'm going to walk you through the stages of your plan here, so don't hesitate to make a start now, even if you're not 100 per cent clear of what you want to achieve. Doing something is always better than doing nothing, and doing something with some structure often helps you find your way by trial and error.

I personally like to physically write and sketch my programmes by hand, but if you prefer to work on a spreadsheet, then take the time to draw something up that you can come back to time and again. If you have never kept a journal or diary of any kind before, it might seem elaborate to detail what you are thinking in relation to your exercise in this way, but once you get the hang of it, a simple plan won't even take you very long, and you can always change it later as your understanding of how to use the information in this book evolves and develops.

Sticking to the plan

There is only one thing that will mess up a good plan, and that's not actually doing it. Changing a plan before you've given it a chance to work its magic is another common pitfall.

In my experience, the most common reason for this is lack of confidence combined with a lack of discipline. Even the best training plan in the world will take some time to adapt to, and in the early stages of training things may get a little worse before they start to get better. Remember that the first stage in Seyle's stress adaption model is '1st alarm'. In practical terms, when you start on a new training plan you are going to feel it, and there will be a stress response in new-found areas of your body that have been unexplored for some time. You won't immediately adapt to what you are doing, and it may feel difficult, both physically and mentally, for the first couple of weeks.

You should expect to feel some discomfort, both with the exercises themselves and with the habit of doing them. When you feel this discomfort, stick to your plan. If you have written down your plan, you can refer back to it time and time again, to remind yourself what you are trying to achieve and how you are going to do it.

Apart from finding it uncomfortable and the discipline needed to develop a new habit, another common reason for falling off a plan is that you find yourself drawn into someone else's. At the same time as you are losing confidence and struggling with self-discipline, if one of your peers seems to be doing something more exciting and interesting you may find yourself hopping onto their plan, which of course is not designed for you, and may be completely inappropriate at worst and distracting at the very least. In almost all circumstances there is no point in re-evaluating your essential conditioning plan until you have spent a full three months working through the exercises. Take the time to choose those that you feel are right for you, based on what you have learned so far, and execute them.

Spend a little quality time evaluating your goals and making a plan. Then stick to it.

 # Making a yearly plan

The first and most important consideration in making an effective conditioning plan is a proper assessment of how much time you have to exercise and how you are going to slice it up. As a cyclist, most of your training time needs to be spent on the bike, but a quarter to a third of the time you are exercising needs to be spent on your essential conditioning (to include appropriate cross-training where applicable). Don't fall into the trap of filling every spare minute with bike riding, leaving no time for any conditioning work. *Quality* training time is what you are after, and that means prioritizing the conditioning time too.

Being realistic about the time you can consistently put into your training is really important at this stage, and the first time that the macrocycle in your periodization becomes relevant. Remember that your macrocycle places your current year of training in relation to the past year and the year ahead. This more global look is important because it will flag up any obviously overambitious goals that will trip you up at the first hurdle.

The basic variables of time and intensity

Let's say, for example, that you want to complete a 150km mountainous sportive this summer, and that to be confident you can achieve that goal you intend to train for 12 hours a week (nine hours on the bike) in the three months preceding your goal event. You want to make sure your back is strong for the climbing (since it sometimes aches on steeper hills) so you're going to include some stretching and core work regularly as part of your preparation.

If you then reflect on how many hours on average you rode in the summer last year, or what the furthest you've ever ridden is, you can consider the time elements of your cycling goal. If you have no experience of mountainous riding at all, another dimension has been thrown into the mix. Next you can review your conditioning status, and note any time you spent consistently on any conditioning, which together will allow you to see whether your cycling performance goal and training process goals are realistic and achievable this current season, or whether you should set an intermediate goal to succeed in the longer term.

Even if you have no experience of coaching or sport at this stage, you can get a simple common-sense grasp of the two main variables you are evaluating here – time or 'volume' of training and 'intensity' or difficulty of the challenge. This same simple evaluation can be applied to your conditioning status too, from a yearly (macrocycle) perspective first, to help shape your seasonal plan thereafter.

Prioritizing conditioning time

Time (volume) and intensity are two important variables when reviewing your conditioning status. Time is fairly obvious and straightforward (though it should be interconnected with your cycling training time). Simple questions you can ask yourself in relation to your conditioning status in this regard are:

- Did you do any off-the-bike conditioning consistently last year?
- How did this balance with the essential conditioning equation of a quarter to a third of total exercise time being an appropriate amount?

These two questions give you an idea of where you are starting from and whether you spent enough time conditioning to balance the amount of time you spent on the bike.

A seasonal evaluation of how much time you are spending on the bike across the seasons will give you some clear direction as to the amount of time you need to spend on your essential conditioning programme. For some riders with no real pain issues or problems, off-the-bike conditioning may be absent during the 'in season', but only if a structured conditioning plan is in place for the remaining nine months of the year. Even for experienced riders in good overall condition, appropriate off-the-bike exercise during the in season will aid recovery and enhance performance.

Intensity in relation to conditioning

To begin to evaluate the intensity – or perhaps more accurately in relation to conditioning exercise, the *quality* – of the conditioning that you put in, you can ask yourself the following questions:

- What type of conditioning did you include and where does it sit across the 'success formula' spectrum? (flexibility, strength or core)
- Did you experience any issues, injuries or difficulties in response to or incidental to any conditioning exercise?
- Did the type of conditioning change throughout the year to complement your cycling training and to allow you to progress?

Some of you will have no consistent conditioning off the bike at this stage, and effectively have a clean slate to make a start this year. Others may have explicitly been working on core exercises or strength exercises, but perhaps only in the 'off season'.

Reviewing your yearly plan

Review your goals for your current macrocycle, or yearly plan, and put them in context of last year, and next year.

Last year ...

In the table below, start first by jotting down the following:

- How much riding you were doing in each of the seasons last year
- What type or intensity of riding you did
- How much conditioning of any kind you were doing in each of the seasons last year

- What type of conditioning it was (can you classify it broadly into stretching, strength and core?)
- Add any notes of injuries or issues you experienced through the year

This coming year ...

Then you can outline what you expect you might need to do to reach your goals this coming year, broadly separating your notes into cycling time and intensity, and conditioning time and quality.

Next year ...

It may be a stretch too far to think further ahead than the coming season, so don't worry if you can't add any detail to this part of the table for now. Even keeping it in mind will help you to begin to think *bigger* in your periodization.

Season	Last year	This year	Next year
Autumn			
Winter			
Spring			
Summer			

If you have experienced injuries or issues with your off-the-bike conditioning in the past, the chances are that you pitched your approach at the wrong level for your conditioning status. For example, if you are very stiff and have a weak core, strength training is likely to cause problems. Alternatively, it may be that the exercises you selected or the way you executed them were not ideal for cyclists.

Both these barriers to progress should be eliminated by the approach taken in this book. However, the more deconditioned you are, the slower you may have to go, and it may take you more than one year to confidently tackle your goals. Often if you have a challenging goal that is outside of your current level of training, making a two- or even three-year plan allows your body to adapt optimally, without overreaching in any way that might cause injury. If you make a plan and keep it, you will know you are moving in the right direction because you will be able to do more of the exercises in this book more easily.

 # Making a seasonal plan

Remembering that your macrocycle view places your current year of conditioning in relation to the past year and the year ahead, adding some detail to your plan throughout the seasons can help it to start to take shape in a more meaningful way. This is where we will start to look at your training in three-monthly blocks.

A breakdown of the time you are likely to spend on the bike and the intensity of your cycling training in any given season (your 'mesocycle') will give shape to your conditioning plan. The time you spend on your conditioning will remain relatively stable at one-third to one-half of the time you spend on the bike. But the nature of the conditioning will change to dovetail with the changing emphasis of your cycling training.

I've started my discussion of my seasonal (three-monthly) plans in the autumn, which for most British and European riders is the time of year when your main cycling activities will be coming to a close. If you are involved in racing or riding sportives, late summer is the time when you should be enjoying the best weather, but when the weather changes and with less events on the calendar, there tends to be a natural pause for you to evaluate your successes and failures, and begin to consider what you might want to do better next year.

If you have been stretching yourself with some new challenges and a full schedule through the summer months, chances are your performance will be starting to decline too, as fatigue sets in and your body begins to need a change or a rest.

In this section I describe each mesocycle in terms of its relationship to your cycling first, so the period which I am referring to as 'in season' will fall in a British calendar summer when your riding will most likely be at its peak. In a way your conditioning plan will have the opposite structure, with the most important season for conditioning being in the 'off season' or winter months, when there can be more intensity in your conditioning programme because it's not there in your cycling training.

Autumn (post-season)

The autumn 'post-season' period is the best time to start to make a training plan, since it allows you a full nine months before the main summer season comes back around, or in view of your conditioning exercises, three months of preparation work before you hit the winter period during which you will want to maximize your off-the-bike gains.

Some cyclists have some time off the bike completely at this time of year, but most will drop the intensity and volume of what they are doing to allow for recovery from the in-season challenges.

It's a good time of year to review your cycling drills and skills, and go back to basics with some fluid, relaxed pedalling, or work on your bike fit and posture so that you have plenty of time to settle into any changes through the winter months.

Even if motivation is low and you are feeling tired, an introduction of conditioning elements as appropriate can give you a welcome change of focus and set you up for the more challenging conditioning work to come later. The post-season is a good time to emphasize flexibility and mobility exercises from Chapter 2 of this book, together with some core exercises from Chapter 3 if appropriate. It can also establish the important habit of putting in the quality time that you will need to see improvements in the long term.

If you are considering including some classes as part of your cross-training in the winter phase, this autumn period is a good time to try out a few of the options too, to find a class that suits you and an instructor or coach that you like.

Winter (off season)

The winter months are the ideal time to make significant headway in terms of your physical condition off the bike, to give you a more robust and adaptable body when you come to the more intense cycling training you will likely want to include in your preseason phase.

Depending on the weather, most cyclists will use this time to develop the aerobic 'base' that underpins any higher-intensity fitness work that will come later. This generally means putting in as much time as is feasible outside, but also using indoor turbo trainers for some heart-rate-based steady-state sessions.

In some instances, when the weather is really bad, the number of hours on the bike simply has to drop, and so the proportionate amount of conditioning time can drift up towards the half rather than the more typical third of the time spent on the bike. Although most cyclists would rather ride outside, this period can be extremely effective for both cycling fitness and conditioning progress. With only 6 or 7 hours on the bike, and 2–2½ hours off it, strength gains in particular can be achieved.

I have found that it's possible to integrate some sport-specific on-the-bike strengthening together with the steady-state aerobic work that predominates for most cyclists during this period. Integrating some 'over-gearing' or seated hill simulations as part of steady-state heart-rate-based sessions can help your brain and body develop muscular strength and endurance at the same time as that all important aerobic fitness.

When on-the-bike strengthening is supported by off-the-bike strength exercises, gains during this period can be significant. Even if your conditioning programme leaves you with some muscle soreness, it's unlikely that this will have any negative impact on the moderate intensity riding that will most likely be the focus on the bike at this time.

If your body is well balanced enough and you have been working on some off-the-bike conditioning for some time, this will be the time of year to focus on the strength essentials outlined in Chapter 3 of this book. Focusing on technique at first but then adding load as soon as you can, you should expect to see significant improvements in the amount of weight you can lift throughout this period.

You may choose to include some key core exercises as you see fit for your personal needs too, but the winter period is the one where you should be working on the exercises as far right on the success formula continuum as your body will allow.

Spring (preseason)

The preseason, or 'early season' as it might be called for some riders who target a full six months throughout the summer, is the time when you want to start to see measurable improvements on the bike. During this period your sport-specific cycling training takes priority again, but that does not mean that your conditioning programme should stop altogether.

Your cycling training at this time will be shaped by your goals for the summer, and may focus on speed and accelerations if you are racing, or threshold fitness and strength endurance if you are looking towards some hilly sportives. The duration and intensity of the efforts will likely be quite specific, but will need more energy and focus as well as needing adequate recovery between sessions.

In terms of strength and power on the bike, drills and skills can be included as part of the more challenging intervals. In my opinion, any out-of-the-saddle work has to be done on the road, such as with standing climbing or sprints and accelerations, which could be a focus here. The higher-intensity seated efforts, whether indoors or outdoors, will need more muscular effort than the more moderate 'tempo' type work too, so it's important that your conditioning work at this time does not leave you with any muscle soreness that detracts from these quality sessions.

For most riders, this will mean taking the strength work out of the programme during the preseason and having more emphasis on the core exercises in Chapter 4 of this book. For some riders, a 'neuro-tonic' approach to the strength work can allow you to maintain a certain amount of the programme a little bit longer. Where a combination of neuro-tonic strength work and core exercises are included during this period, it will be easier to pick up your conditioning programme at a higher level at the end of the season.

A neuro-tonic approach to strength work is one where you include enough of an exercise to stimulate the nervous system without causing significant fatigue in the muscles. There are several ways to use this approach effectively. You can maintain the intensity or 'load' of the exercise, but reduce the number of repetitions or sets so that you stop before fatigue sets in. For some riders, it might be best to work for 6–8 reps of your 10–12 rep load. For others, one full set (instead of 2–3) might work better. If you are familiar with the strength components of your programme and confident about your form, you can work with a lighter load and higher repetition range in a continuous circuit, maintaining the movement patterns in the minimum time and with the minimum muscular fatigue.

Summer (in season)

The in season is what you have been waiting for and the time you should expect to see your best performances on the bike and the fruits of your labours for the previous nine months. If you have dovetailed your cycling training with your conditioning effectively, everything should come together during the summer so that you are feeling strong and fast on the bike, without any injuries or issues, even with your hardest, most challenging riding.

Quite simply, you should be doing all the riding you want during the peak of your season, taking in the goals that you have set and enjoying the best of the weather whenever you can.

If you have no injury problems and feel confident of your conditioning status, this is the time of year when some riders can afford to let their conditioning programme drop off altogether. If you want to make the most of your riding, you will want to borrow back that precious time you've spent on your conditioning and use it on longer days in the saddle.

With a structured plan the rest of the year, and with no injuries or issues, it's possible to let your off-the-bike conditioning drop during the in season. However, most riders, and especially those with a history of injuries or issues, do better by maintaining some stretching or core maintenance exercises to enhance recovery and maintain postural alignment.

Typical seasonal schedule and adaptations

Season	On-the-bike emphasis	Off-the-bike conditioning
Autumn (post-season)	Rest and recovery (postural correction, bike fit review)	Establishing habits, flexibility and mobility development with some core
Winter (off season)	Aerobic base building (seated strength drills)	Strength development with core progressions
Spring (preseason)	Event-specific higher-intensity intervals (standing and seated accelerations and sprints)	Neuro-tonic strength maintenance and core emphasis
Summer (in season)	Optimal cycling performance	Stretching and core maintenance, recovery emphasis

Remembering the success formula – personalizing your approach

The broad plan outlined above gives you an idea of what your conditioning programme could look like across the seasons. However, there is plenty of scope for personalization so that your essential conditioning programme meets your individual needs, particularly if the plan above is too comprehensive for you to get your head round.

Hopefully by working through this book, and in particular by trying some of the exercises in Chapters 2–4, you have some idea whether flexibility, strength or core needs to be your main priority, and where you sit along the success formula spectrum.

Ideally, your conditioning plan would include all three elements as you progress through the seasons as outlined above. However, for some riders an emphasis on two aspects may be more effective, particularly if you have no experience of consistent conditioning at all and are overwhelmed by the prospect of learning so many new exercises.

For example, if you start with a flexibility-focused programme you will hopefully progress to include some core elements in your schedule as you change from one season to the next. If you start with a core-focused plan, you may include some strength elements as your alignment improves and you feel ready to include some of the primal pattern movements. There is enough scope within the variety of exercises in this book to work in this way for as long as you want, changing the exercises you have chosen from each section as you move through the phases of your year.

Below I have outlined two alternative schedules for you to adopt if you recognize yourself in the following descriptions:

Alternative schedule A uses exercises from Chapters 2 and 4 only on stretching and core essentials

Adopt this schedule below if:

- you have a pattern of injury associated with muscle strains, joint sprains or lumbar disc problems
- you know that you are very stiff and have poor posture
- you have not done any consistent conditioning of any kind for several years.

Alternative schedule A

Season	On-the-bike emphasis	Off-the-bike conditioning
Autumn (post-season)	Rest and recovery (postural correction, bike fit review)	Establishing habits, flexibility and mobility development (both pre-exercise stretching and post-exercise stretching)
Winter (off season)	Aerobic base building (seated strength drills)	Pre-exercise stretching and selected core exercises (focus on stability/postural variations with longer holds)
Spring (preseason)	Event-specific higher-intensity intervals (standing and seated accelerations and sprints)	Pre-exercise stretching and selected core exercises (focus on strength variations with 8–12 rep range)
Summer (in season)	Optimal cycling performance	Pre-exercise stretching and selected core maintenance (focus on stability/postural variations with longer holds)

Alternative schedule B uses exercises from Chapters 3 and 4 only

Adopt alternative schedule B if:

- You have a history of injury associated with instability, subluxations and things 'going out'
- You know that you are hypermobile
- You are a female rider
- You have not done any consistent conditioning of any kind for several years

Alternative schedule B

Season	On-the-bike emphasis	Off-the-bike conditioning
Autumn (post-season)	Rest and recovery (postural correction, bike fit review)	Selected core exercises (focus on Swiss ball variations)
Winter (off season)	Aerobic base building (seated strength drills)	Strength development with some core maintenance
Spring (preseason)	Event-specific higher-intensity intervals (standing, and seated accelerations and sprints)	Strength development with some core maintenance
Summer (in season)	Optimal cycling performance	Neuro-tonic strength maintenance with core maintenance

Reviewing your seasonal plan

Using the templates and guidelines outlined, now sketch out your own seasonal plan. You may have goals or aspects to your year that make your plan different from those I've used above so I've left the season parts for you to fill in yourself, in case your goal events are at a different time of year. The principles remain the same. Just shift the timing to peak in your 'in season'.

Season	On-the-bike emphasis	Off-the-bike conditioning
(post-season)		
(off season)		
(preseason)		
(in season)		

Making a weekly plan

Once you have fleshed out your mesocycle view for the current season, it's time to get into the nitty gritty of what a week of training will look like for the next three months (your *micro*cycle). The detail of your weekly plan will fall into place more easily when you have been through the process of your yearly and monthly plans first, and often it's easier to focus day to day on what you want to get done when you have this perspective on where it fits into the whole.

As always, you should start with your riding schedule, and most people do better with a weekly pattern to their cycling training. Once you have sketched out the time you are spending on the bike, it makes sense to put into place any other time commitments that are regular and fixed, and make training impossible. You would probably include work hours, family time and any other regular commitments that rule out exercise.

One thing to bear in mind at this stage is that no one knows what will work best for you better than you. There really are as many ways to make your conditioning plan effective as there are people, but what you have to ensure is that you find a way to regularly put the time in.

Some people like to get up early to stretch and train before work. Others like to get to the gym at lunchtime to get a break from the office, and others still have the best chance of exercise in the evening when the kids have gone to bed. Some riders like to bolt their pre-stretching and core work on to their turbo training, stretching beforehand and working through the core exercise immediately afterwards. Some people like to do two or three longer sessions a week without having to do anything in between, while others like to do a bit of something every day. It really is up to you to choose your own adventure.

At this stage, jotting down some idea of when you will do some conditioning and roughly what type will be helpful.

Example weekly review

This schedule represents 12–13 hours of riding (including commutes), with three hours of conditioning (1 hour 40 minutes of stretching and 1 hour 20 minutes of core work). It has a stretching and core focus.

Example week

Time	Mon	Tue	Wed	Thur	Fri	Sat	Sun
7am	Pre-stretching 10 mins	Pre-stretching 10 mins		Pre-stretching 10 mins	Pre-stretching 10 mins		Pre-stretching 20 mins
8	Cycling commute	Cycling commute		Cycling commute	Cycling commute	Football with kids	Endurance ride on road
9	WORK						
10							
11							
12pm							
1							
2	WORK						
3						Pre-stretch + 40 min core (A&B)	Food shop, family time
4			School				
5	Cycling commute		pick up	Cycling commute	Cycling commute		
6	10 mins pre-stretch + Turbo training			10 mins pre-stretch + turbo training			
7	20 mins core A		20 mins stretching	20 mins core B	Date night		
8							

YOUR typical week of cycling, life and conditioning time

Time	Mon	Tue	Wed	Thur	Fri	Sat	Sun
7am							
8							
9							
10							
11							
12pm							
1							
2							
3							
4							
5							
6							
7							
8							

Where to place key cross-training activities

The example does not include any of the cross-training activities discussed in Chapter 5. A lunchtime swim or Pilates class would be a good addition to this programme if these options were appealing, and would allow my example cyclist to drop the longer stretching programme and perhaps one of the core programmes from the weekly schedule.

It's important to plan any cross-training activities on a weekly basis to ensure that you progress with the activity as part of your broader programme. Making a commitment to a regular class or session is important, since if you miss it you may not meet your conditioning time quota.

Using time-based templates to design your own conditioning programme

For your weekly plan to be most effective, the time considerations are once again the starting point. This will make it most likely that you will stick to the plan, to ensure that you make the progress you deserve. I have included some conditioning templates here that slice your conditioning plan into 10, 20, 30 and 40-minute schedules to give you as much flexibility as possible in designing your own programme.

Ten minutes doesn't seem very long, but in some instances breaking up the time you condition into these manageable chunks can make significant changes to the balance of your body. A conditioning programme with a strong emphasis on stretching, for example, can be built on frequent 10-minute pre-exercise stretching programmes (before every bike ride, for example, or daily in the morning), coupled with longer, more developmental stretching in the evenings before bed. Creating a more developmental stretch programme simply involves using the same stretches for longer and adding the 'post-exercise only' variations that you will see in Chapter 2.

Frequent short bouts of 10 minutes of 'pre-stretching' almost daily, coupled with longer, more developmental stretch sessions of 20–30 minutes two or three times a week, can be an effective way to become more flexible.

Core-focused programmes can largely be built on 20–30-minute sessions, and they may need to be made up of several different variations that cover all the exercises that you want to include. If you are time squeezed during the week, you could look to include a longer programme at the weekend and then split it into two parts Monday to Friday (so that you manage two shorter sessions in the week), so that you get all the exercises in your programme twice a week.

Short core sessions of 20–30 minutes, including two or three exercises for three to four sets, can be an effective way to develop your core strength by including four or five sessions a week. In this instance you might design two mini-programmes that you alternate and if you have time for a longer session bolt them both together. By changing the emphasis from stability (longer hold) and strength (8–12 rep range) exercises, as well as including different dimensions (sagittal, frontal or transverse plane focus) you will allow your body to adapt between sessions and develop your core stability and strength in three dimensions.

More comprehensive or strength-focused conditioning programmes that require multiple sets and six to eight strength and core exercises might need a full 40-minute session to maximize the benefits. In general, a 40-minute programme will be more effective when the emphasis is on strength and core exercises, because you can have days in between without any conditioning work to allow your muscles to adapt and respond to the movements. Additional elements could be supplemented too (such as pre-ride or post-ride stretching for 10 minutes at a time).

In general terms, the more to the right on the success formula you are working, the more effective longer programmes will be because they will allow enough time for multiple sets, and for recovery between sessions for your body to adapt to the more strength-focused training stimulus. These longer sessions with more of a strength focus will be more intense and time consuming, but would only need to be included in your schedule two or three times a week to be effective.

Based on these basic ideas, I have drawn up some example schedules for you to work with to sketch out your own programmes. Have a look over them now, and if you are ready, copy a few so that you can sketch out your ideas.

Using the conditioning templates

In the templates that follow, each box represents two minutes. Most of the exercises in this book can be completed in two minutes, allowing for the rest between sets. There are a few exceptions, notably the stability and postural core exercises, which may take four minutes per set to work through. List your chosen exercises in the left-hand column, leaving the extra rows (time) needed for completing multiple sets.

In working through the chapters of this book, and in consideration of your mesocycle emphasis (i.e. what the focus of your programme is at this time), choose 10–20 exercises in total that you want to include in your programme. Then separate them out into the divided (A and B, for example) programmes as you have chosen how to slice them up.

Any programme including all elements (stretch, strength and core) should be included in the order of pre-stretches, strength exercises and then core exercises. Any post-exercise stretches should be done at the end of the programme. If a programme includes only two elements, the order remains the same, the third element is just taken out. So strength and core exercises would be done in that order. Pre-stretching and core exercises will be performed in that order too.

If in practice when you work through the exercises it takes a bit less time than you expected, you can always add more exercises, but I've taken this approach to encourage you to design manageable programmes that you can do within the time allowed.

The essential conditioning templates

10-minute pre-stretching template

Name of the exercise	Number of repetitions/notes	Weight/ load record
Stretch 1		
Stretch 2		
Stretch 3		
Stretch 4		
Stretch 5		

20-minute post-exercise stretching template

Name of the exercise	Number of repetitions/notes	Weight/ load record
Stretch 1 (spinal mobilization)		
– spend 4 mins total		
Stretch 2 (spinal mobilization)		
– spend 4 mins total		
Stretch 3		
Stretch 4		
Stretch 5		
Stretch 6		
Stretch 7		
Stretch 8		

20-minute core-focused template

Name of the exercise	Number of repetitions/notes	Weight/ load record
Pre-stretch 1		
Pre-stretch 2		
Pre-stretch 3		
Core exercise 1 – set 1		
– set 2		
– set 3		
Core exercise 2 – set 1		
– set 2		
– set 3		
Post-exercise stretch		

30-minute core-focused template

Name of the exercise	Number of repetitions/notes	Weight/ load record
Pre-stretch 1		
Pre-stretch 2		
Core exercise 1 – set 1		
– set 2		
– set 3		
Core exercise 2 – set 1		
– set 2		
– set 3		
Core exercise 3 – set 1		
– set 2		
– set 3		
Strength exercise 1 – set 1		
– set 2		
– set 3		

40-minute strength (and core) session template

Name of the exercise	Number of repetitions/notes	Weight/ load record
Pre-stretch 1		
Pre-stretch 2		
Pre-stretch 2		
Strength exercise 1 – set 1		
– set 2		
– set 3		
Strength exercise 2 – set 1		
– set 2		
– set 3		
Strength exercise 3 – set 1		
– set 2		
– set 3		
Strength exercise 4 – set 1		
– set 2		

40-minute strength (and core) session template (cont.)

Name of the exercise	Number of repetitions/notes	Weight/ load record
– set 3		
Core exercise 1 – set 1		
– set 2		
Core exercise 2 – set 1		
– set 2		

References

Chek, P. (2004) *How to Eat, Move and Be Healthy!* CHEK Institute.

Gracovetsky, S. (1988) *The Spinal Engine.* Springer-Verlag.

Magee, D. J. (2008) *Orthopaedic Physical Assessment*, 5th edition. Saunders.

Page, P., Frank, C. C. and Lardner, R. (2010) *Assessment and Treatment of Muscle Imbalances: The Janda Approach.* Human Kinetics.

Index

dumbbell 117–18, 149
  preparation 115–16, 149
disc bulge/herniation 42
drills 230–1
dumbbells 12, 13
  bent-over row 139, 150
  dead lift 117–18, 149
  front-loaded split squat 123, 149
  front-loaded squats 113, 148
  Swiss ball chest press 131–2, 150
  Swiss ball seated shoulder press 133–4,
    150

endurance 21, 218–20
equipment 13
exercise classes 237–45
extension with rotation 181
external oblique 164

fascia 46
flat back 48, 114
flexibility 34, 38, 218–20
flexion dominance 26, 44, 185
foam roller mobilization
  horizontal 53–4, 89
  iliotibial band 68–9
  longitudinal 50–2, 89
foam rollers 12, 13, 49
footwear for cross-training 229
form principle 101, 192
front crawl 232
functional strength 22–3

gait 31
general conditioning 23–31

gluteals 63, 67, 108, 160–2
goals 252–4
group exercise classes 237–45

hamstrings
  cycling prime movers 63
  lack of flexibility in 30
  squats and 108
  stretches 73–82, 90–1
  tightness in 46, 55
  weakness in 160–2
hip flexors 70–2
hips and legs stretches/mobilizations
  63–82
horizontal foam roller mobilization 53–4,
  89
horse stances 187–90, 211
human movement 17, 21
hypermobility 159, 239

iliotibial band (ITB) 46
  foam roller mobilization 68–9, 90
  iliotibial band syndrome 68
indoor games 235–6
injuries 14, 18–19, 30, 220
instability 157
intensity variable 256–7
internal oblique 164
isolated exercises 29–30
isometric exercises 170

kneeling plank 195–6, 212

legs *see* hips and legs stretches/
  mobilizations

lifting 26

longitudinal foam roller mobilization 50–2, 89

lower back 42, 55–8, 61–2, 114, 160

lower body Russian twist 203–7, 212–13

lumbar spine 42, 55–8, 61–2, 114, 160

lunge *see* split squat

lunging 21, 27–8

    see also split squat

McKenzie press-up 57–8, 89

motivation 252–3

muscle(s)

    shortness 103–4

    soreness 32

    upper body and neck 44–5

    see also individual exercises; individual muscles

neck 43, 83–8, 135

neck crunch 199, 212

neural inhibition 65

neuro-tonic approach 263

neutral spine philosophy 101–2, 167

pain 14, 18–19

paired sports 235–6

passive doorframe hamstring stretch 82

pec stretch 50–2

periodization 221, 248

Pilates 240–2

piriformis stretch 64–6, 90

piriformis syndrome 64

plank on toes 196

planks 192–9, 211–12

planning

    benefits of 252

    guidelines 252–5

    importance of 250–2

    problems with lack of 251

    science behind 248

    seasonal plan 259–68

    training cycles 249

    weekly plan 269–79

    yearly plan 255–9

positional problem areas 41–5

post-exercise stretches 59–60

posture 19, 41–5, 167–9, 208–9, 213

pre-exercise stretches 59–60

press-up 127–30

    full 130, 150

    kneeling 129, 149

    plank preparation 127–8, 149

primal patterns/fitness 17, 21, 22, 98

prime movers 107, 124

prone cobra 176–80, 210

pulling 21, 29–30

pulling exercises 135–41

pull-ups 29

pushing 21, 28

pushing exercises 124–34

quadriceps 46, 63, 70–2, 108

quadriceps dominance 161

racket sports 235–6

reciprocal inhibition 64

rectus abdominus 164

rectus femoris 70

rehabilitation 220

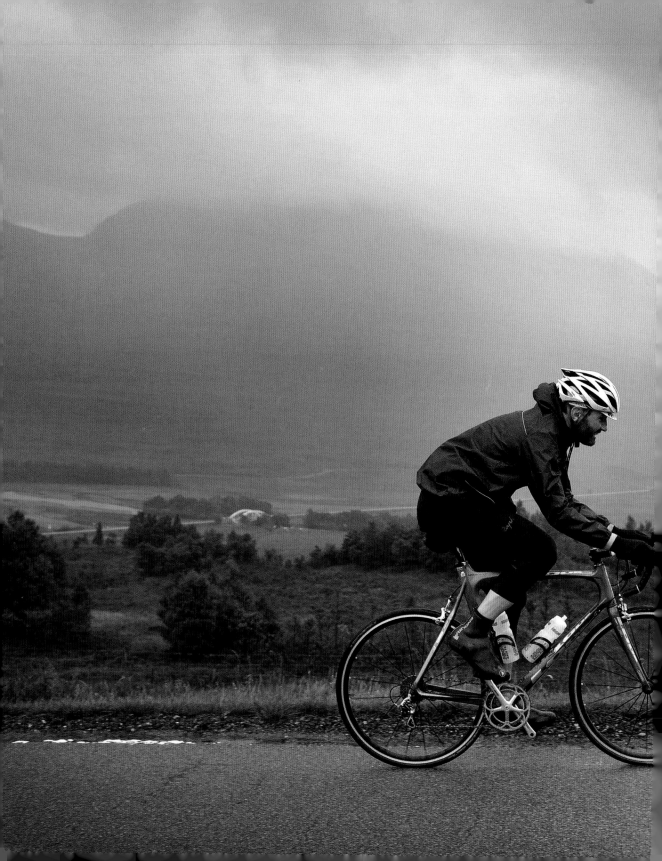

Remember the
success formula:

FLEXIBILITY
+ CORE STABILITY
+ STRENGTH
= POWER POTENTIAL